Forensic Medicine - The Role of Current Technology in Forensic Medicine and Forensic Sciences

Edited by Kamil Hakan Dogan

Published in London, United Kingdom

Forensic Medicine - The Role of Current Technology in Forensic Medicine and Forensic Sciences
http://dx.doi.org/10.5772/intechopen.1004672
Edited by Kamil Hakan Dogan

Contributors
Asma Jan Muhammad, Dodany Machado Mendoza, Hiroshi Kinoshita, Kamil Hakan Dogan, Nihal Yetimoğlu, Praveen Kumar Pradhan, Sella Takei, Takehiko Murase

Notice

Statements and opinions expressed in the chapters are these of the individual contributors and not necessarily those of the editors or publisher. No responsibility is accepted for the accuracy of information contained in the published chapters. The publisher assumes no responsibility for any damage or injury to persons or property arising out of the use of any materials, instructions, methods or ideas contained in the book.

First published in London, United Kingdom, 2025 by IntechOpen
IntechOpen is the global imprint of INTECHOPEN LIMITED, registered in England and Wales, registration number: 11086078, 167-169 Great Portland Street, London, W1W 5PF, United Kingdom

For EU product safety concerns: IN TECH d.o.o., Prolaz Marije Krucifikse Kozulić 3, 51000 Rijeka, Croatia, info@intechopen.com or visit our website at intechopen.com.

British Library Cataloguing-in-Publication Data
A catalogue record for this book is available from the British Library

Forensic Medicine - The Role of Current Technology in Forensic Medicine and Forensic Sciences
Edited by Kamil Hakan Dogan
p.cm.
Print ISBN 978-1-83634-650-0
Online ISBN 978-1-83634-649-4
eBook (PDF) ISBN 978-1-83634-651-7

If disposing of this product, please recycle the paper responsibly.

IntechOpen

intechopen.com

Built by scientists, for scientists

Meet the editor

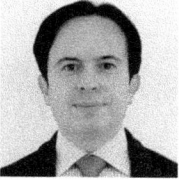

Kamil Hakan Dogan MD, Ph.D. is a Full Professor and Chair in the Department of Forensic Medicine at Selcuk University, Faculty of Medicine in Türkiye. Dr. Dogan received his MD from Gazi University, Faculty of Medicine in 2000. Following his extensive research in the field of forensic medicine, he earned his Ph.D. in Biochemistry in 2012. He gives lectures on Forensic Medicine and Medical Ethics to medical students as well as students of the dentistry and law faculties. He is the editor of eight books and a reviewer for several international journals, and he has published over 200 articles in refereed journals, chapters in textbooks and abstracts in scientific meetings. His publications have been cited over 1,000 times.

Contents

Preface

As we experience rapid changes in science and technology, the fields of forensic and medical sciences are at a vital point where innovation, ethical reflection, and practical use converge. The use of modern tools and approaches in both investigative and clinical areas not only reshapes our processes for uncovering truth and providing justice but also challenges the foundations of our conventional moral and legal standards.

The book entitled *Forensic Medicine – The Role of Current Technology in Forensic Medicine and Forensic Sciences* brings together a compelling collection of chapters that explore the multifaceted developments shaping these dynamic fields. From the rapid advancements in DNA examination to the intricate contributions of forensic dentistry, every aspect delves deeply into specialized yet interconnected themes.

Through the study of aircraft tragedies using forensic anthropology, experts highlight the significant role that human remains play in uncovering vital information about some of the most severe occurrences. The implementation of energy-dispersive X-ray fluorescence spectrometry (EDX) in the study of foreign entities showcases the expansion of non-invasive elemental analysis within the field of forensic investigation. Alongside these technological innovations, there is a crucial and reflective inquiry into medical ethics, compelling us to rethink the core principles that underpin our healthcare systems as we face the dilemmas associated with artificial intelligence and end-of-life decisions.

When combined, these chapters weave a detailed account that is intellectually challenging and useful in practical contexts. This resource is beneficial for a diverse audience, including forensic scientists, medical practitioners, ethicists, legal specialists, and students, offering essential insights and thoughtful perspectives on the challenges of modern professional practice.

In light of advancing technologies and shifting societal demands, the most effective tools we possess are our principles of honesty, our adaptability, and our firm dedication to the dignity of every individual. We aim for this book to stimulate dialogue, enhance cooperation across diverse areas of study, and significantly contribute to the ongoing fight for justice and ethical care in a world that is growing increasingly complex.

With determination and respect, we should persist in progressing in the forensic and medical fields, grounded in both creativity and moral accountability.

Kamil Hakan Dogan
Department of Forensic Medicine,
Selcuk University Faculty of Medicine,
Konya, Türkiye

Chapter 1

Introductory Chapter: The Role of Current Technology in Forensic Medicine and Forensic Sciences

Kamil Hakan Dogan

1. Introduction

Part of the rules and functions of the branch of science and expertise called forensic science and medicine include evidence collection, storage, and evaluation; evaluation of the personality and relation of a person by evaluating the corpse, how he died, when he died, and where he died; and aiding law enforcement authorities to catch the perpetrator in the determination and verification of the level of the wound, to identify the hidden and evident traumas in the body, and to gather physical evidence left at the crime scene. Technology is playing a bigger role in making these duties easier and more exact. Rapid improvements in medicine have been transformed into its legitimate branches, such as forensic science and medicine. Physicochemical methods are frequently used in forensic science and expertise in routine experiments. Studies mainly focus on the development of new techniques to be used in forensic laboratories. Current technologies that aid forensic science and expertise in criminal investigations are summarized. Some techniques include DNA printing, body scans, toxicology, and pointcut analysis as well as chemometrics. The future developments and obstructions of technological advances are also discussed [1, 2].

2. Overview of forensic medicine and forensic sciences

2.1 Definition and scope

Rapid progress has been made in the last few decades in human civilization and other areas with the aid of advances in the field of technology. The development of technology in information, medicine, electronics, legal rules, etc., has a significant effect on various sciences, especially in the area of forensic sciences. Forensic sciences and auxiliary techniques have a specific place throughout the judicial process. Today, solutions are being found for many criminal acts with the aid of these sciences. Each crime can be considered unique. Criminalistic history has utilized tools of the present period in the examination and solution of most crimes. The discovery of the very first fingerprint, X-ray, and other tests, as well as the highly developed physical and electronic devices utilized in the examination of toxic, chemical, and radiological content, has not just made criminalistic examination a significant source of punishment,

IntechOpen

but also serves as a significant deterrent for potential criminals. Those responsible for the planning of some crimes may avoid the risk of punishment thanks to the use of these devices [3, 4].

2.2 Historical development

The historical development of technological mechanisms to enhance forensic sciences is a start in gaining an understanding of the general field of forensic sciences and technologies. Documented forensic sciences date back to at least 1248 and 1249 A.D. when two Chinese poems were located. These poems presented the use of entomology to determine the post-mortem interval of two children's corpses by examining the presence of fly eggs. Many procedures for evaluating evidence can be traced from the procedure of publicly showing physical evidence in a courtroom and yesterday's collection of a DNA sample to today's pass/fail or "yes" and "no" output. Depending on the operational definition of a technology, one technology might appear at different points in our standardized timeline. For example, the microscope might appear as one developmental technology, bypassing all of its improvements and applications during a long period of time, without any hint of the computer but appearing later in the developmental timeline, suggesting a punctuated appearance in our records based on failures to define the technology we are attempting to track [5, 6].

3. Importance of technology in forensic investigations

3.1 Enhanced evidence collection and analysis

The speed and precision benefits and risks of high-throughput DNA sequencing, high-throughput data analysis, and amplification techniques are according to their forensic application. The integration of different strategies may lead forensic protocols to accommodate the identification of single traces or use the low copy number requirements. The correct balance is between the conservational implications of performing ultra-deep SNP genotyping and the potential information produced to contribute to minimizing the size of DNA databases for forensic purposes. The investigation of somatic changes in DNA requires increasing the detection limit of forensically relevant SNPs, to the extent that genotype concordance decreases. Results bring new insights to the limits of the power of predicting eye color. Finally, the QC procedures do not exert a predictable effect on allele balance. Difficult single-nucleotide polymorphism (SNP) genotyping is performed at low DNA input levels [7].

3.2 Advancements in DNA profiling

Traditional methods of DNA profiling that use RFLPs, minisatellite restriction fragment length polymorphism typing, and PCR-based typing systems yield results that, while extremely significant in genetic terms, may yield limited results from evidence samples. Low copy number or trace DNA refers to the profile that might be obtained from clothing or tools that have been handled by suspects or individuals present at a crime scene. When DNA is extracted from an evidence sample, and only a limited number of cells from one of the cells are carried out, this raises the possibility of signal-to-noise ratios and the potential for the admixed profiles of others. Profiling efforts using these types of samples can result in muddy or blurred profiles or in the lack of any information capable of being employed in database searches. This prevents the interrogation from potentially including whatever reference profile information might be available. The problems in the enucleation necessary for DNA extraction from particularly ancient and moribund cells can also be equally problematic.

PCR-based techniques were introduced 1 year after the first use of PCR in the field of DNA fingerprinting. There have been vast improvements in technology since then. Notable among these was the introduction of capillary electrophoresis. Replacing the slab gels and current electrophoresis tanks used, which were constructed of glass or polyacrylamide, with fused silica tubing with an internal coating of polyacrylamide resulted in great advantages. It was no longer necessary to handle glass plates, and increasing throughput was allowed for by reducing run times and miniaturizing the gel matrices. The capacity now to add more sulfonic rinse dye-labeled primer pairs to the mixture and analyze several loci at one time has provided more reliable results and more data. With new gene amplification real-time detection technologies, scientists can achieve increased sensitivity. Two common applications of effective PCR include quantification and quality control [5].

4. Key technological innovations in forensic medicine and forensic sciences

4.1 Digital forensics

Digital forensics refers to forensic science pertaining to evidence found in digital storage media and is often used in the investigation of computer systems and data, that is, computer devices containing digital evidence. Digital forensics typically involves the recovery and analysis of material found on personal and business-related electronic devices, which can be in the form of credit card information, intellectual property, proprietary information, or a myriad of other forms that were purposefully erased or unknowingly removed from a subject or victim and then possibly electronically sent or distributed excessively. Digital forensics can also be utilized to work backwards to identify a specific perpetrator of a crime. Digital forensics is frequently utilized in both civil and criminal cases and has become significant for many medical and health professionals due to the escalating occurrences of cyberbullying, blackmail, slander, and malfeasance cases relative to the healthcare industry. These cases are becoming not only more widespread but also in closer proximity such that forensic investigators are frequently consulted to use advanced forensic software programs to assist in identifying an account or individual perpetrating these unethical acts. Digital evidence discovered is important to the legal process as it can pinpoint that an event has occurred, when it occurred, and if any criminal activity has occurred. The main aspect of the digital forensic process is maintaining a documented, secure chain of evidence. In order to verify the integrity of evidence in a computer investigation, we must regularly document and validate its integrity as well as observe and secure continuous succession of custodianship [7].

4.2 Biometrics and facial recognition

The boundaries of studies on biometrics and facial recognition are medical ethics, privacy, tracking systems, verification experiments, skin pigmentation, forensic science, forensic medicine, evidence on the death process and criminal investigation [7].

Studies on facial recognition and biometrics cover an important area for the use of current technology in forensic medicine and forensic sciences. In this chapter, we have tried to describe some technological tools to develop the work of forensic medicine and forensic sciences, although these are not all the technologies available for this field of work. The immense need for forensic science experts to provide accurate, precise, and up-to-date evaluations to the justice system always raises the issue and the dilemma of being able to optimize the work they carry out, along with the many tests they have to perform with all the other possible tools at their disposal. The innovations provided by technology therefore represent an opportunity that must be valued and adequately assimilated [5].

Technology is making vast strides in various sectors, including the judiciary. The research activity currently carried out involves the integrated use of various disciplines and sectors of technological development. The skin color problem also concerns the so-called skin pigmentation feature, which is an important discriminant. In fact, the color of the irises and the color of the skin are closely related. This relationship must be exploited to obtain useful information for the development of biometric systems, in addition to extracting other important information for the forensic medical field; user privacy must always be safeguarded. In the present work, we evaluated a new methodology that allowed us to non-invasively extract the skin pigment information from iris images for use in biometric systems; we have performed a verification experiment of the obtained information, and the results are very encouraging [8].

5. Challenges and ethical considerations

Advances in the development of portable forensic devices promise a broad application and information sharing. Rapid examination, portability, lightweight, non-invasive techniques, low power consumption, and multimodal functions are important features for the development of a dual-use device in the civil and defense fields. Dual-use technology devices that can trace portable samples, including chemical agent proliferation, should have a standard qualification. Artificial intelligence applications can help the comprehensive analysis of the obtained forensic data and contribute to preventing human errors; however, the failure of computers in practical intelligence raises several ethical, moral, and technical questions regarding the development of the computational capabilities of artificial intelligence, which must be thoroughly studied and addressed. There is a need for the development of international technological standards for the uniform identification and qualification, as well as the sharing and disclosure of forensic data [6].

Moreover, artificial intelligence must respect human rights and freedoms and be based on the principles that guarantee such respect and the other principles for which it is sought. The major challenge of forensic medicine development refers to the incorporation of information technology in the practice of forensic examination, ensuring the appropriate training and qualification of the staff involved, as well as the development and sharing of common, stable, and universally accepted standards and ethical rules. It is very important to research and study computer models in a deep and cautious way, with respect to the sharing and disclosure of forensic data, as well as to assure the right of individuals to make inferences about themselves and others [5].

6. Future trends and implications

The role of current technology in forensic medicine and forensic sciences is a matter of great importance in order to be able to predict future trends and implications efficiently. It remains clear from the discussion made in previous chapters that forensic medicine is not just fixing bones or putting pieces of flesh of the injured body together. The role of a forensic expert in a medico-legal case is not only curing, repairing, and assembling torn-off body parts of the injured bodies. With all respect to the loyalty and wisdom of Florence Nightingale and Hippocrates, a modern forensic expert, when dealing with medico-legal cases, must be possessing both the skills of pain treatment and solving the enigma of crime.

Indeed, there is a multi-disciplinary science designed to aid crime solving through the technological application of scientific knowledge: forensic science. Forensic science, a sub-branch of forensic medicine, uses modern technology (our concern) to examine and compare physical evidence to solve a crime. The reason forensic science exists is to give identification of an unknown suspect and to aid in the prosecution of that person in the commission of a crime. Currently, the scope of forensic science is diverse and has a wide range of possible applications in collecting and examining evidence, tracking criminals, handling cybercrime, and the field of DNA forensics for identifying bodies and the dead. This chapter discusses technological advancements and implications for forensic sciences and the adoption of health informatics techniques for supporting digital criminal evidence preservation.

Author details

Kamil Hakan Dogan
Selcuk University Faculty of Medicine, Konya, Turkey

*Address all correspondence to: drhakan2000@gmail.com

IntechOpen

References

[1] Spellman BA, Eldridge H, Bieber P. Challenges to reasoning in forensic science decisions. Forensic Science International: Synergy. 2021;**4**:100200. DOI: 10.1016/j.fsisyn.2021.100200

[2] Chango X, Flor-Unda O, Gil-Jiménez P, Gómez-Moreno H. Technology in forensic sciences: Innovation and precision. Technologies. 2024;**12**(8):120. DOI: 10.3390/technologies12080120

[3] Alketbi SK. The role of DNA in forensic science: A comprehensive review. International Journal of Science and Research Archive. 2023;**09**(02):814-829. DOI: 10.2139/ssrn.4550489

[4] Roux C, Willis S, Weyermann C. Shifting forensic science focus from means to purpose: A path forward for the discipline? Science & Justice. 2021;**61**(6):678-686. DOI: 10.1016/j.scijus.2021.08.005

[5] Liao Y. Song Ci, the Xi Yuan Ji Lu, and the judicial examination system. In: Jiang X, editor. The High Tide of Science and Technology Development in China. History of Science and Technology in China. Singapore: Springer; 2021. DOI: 10.1007/978-981-15-7847-2_7

[6] Durkin A. Estimating a face: What predicting appearance from DNA reveals about the need to regulate genetic investigations. Washington University Law Review. 2023;**101**:1241

[7] Liritzis I, Boyatzis S, Polymeris GS, Panagopoulou A, Sideris A, Rapti S, et al. Remarks and caution on finds of Kastrouli Mycenaean settlement (loofah, charcoal, bone, wall burnt clay coating, ceramic). Scientific Culture. 2023;**9**(2):1-28. DOI: 10.5281/zenodo.7460006

[8] Almugren KS, Nawi SM, Sabtu SN, Saifunazif AA, Almajid HF, Shafiqah AS, et al. Structural and retrospective bio-dosimetric study of gamma-irradiated human fingernails. Radiation Physics and Chemistry. 2024;**223**:111983. DOI: 10.1016/j.radphyschem.2024.111983

Chapter 2

Revolutionizing DNA Analysis: The Impact of Rapid DNA Sequencing on Modern Forensic Investigations

Asma Jan Muhammad

Abstract

This chapter explains how fast DNA sequencing is revolutionizing forensic science and making the process of criminal investigations much more accurate and efficient. The evolution of DNA analysis tools has made the identification of individuals connected to crime cases significantly easier. With real-time DNA profiling, rapid sequencing cuts processing times from days to hours, making it highly useful in time-sensitive situations. Examples such as solving cold cases, identifying disaster victims, and analyzing crime scenes exemplify the revolutionary potential. The chapter also discusses the challenges in integrating rapid DNA sequencing into forensic work-flows, such as data security, privacy, and ethical implications. These challenges raise the need for strong protocols and guidelines to ensure responsible use. Despite these challenges, rapid sequencing holds great promise for advancing modern criminal justice systems, offering faster and more reliable solutions to longstanding investigative challenges. This chapter underlines how bridging technology and forensic science can help shape the future of criminal investigations to foster a more effective and just legal system by bridging this gap.

Keywords: DNA analysis, rapid DNA sequencing, forensic investigations, criminal identification, criminal forensic science technology

1. Introduction

1.1 Overview of DNA analysis in forensics

DNA analysis has revolutionized forensic science, which revolutionizes the solving of criminal cases and mysteries. DNA is a very reliable source of evidence since no two people are alike except for identical twins. Since its discovery in the 1980s, DNA analyses has been used to link suspects to crime scenes, exonerate wrongly accused people, and solve cold cases [1, 2]. However, conventional methods often take too long and therefore delay justice in critical investigations.

1.2 Importance of rapid DNA sequencing

Rapid DNA sequencing is presently a rising innovation wherein analysis can be conducted in hours instead of days or weeks. It has moreover incredibly progressed the productivity in investigations, subsequently making police decisions faster to avoid even the potential casualty. Being a combination of progressed strategy and innovation, fast DNA sequencing gives results much more rapidly and precisely than forensic science [2, 3].

This chapter addresses the effect of fast DNA sequencing on forensic examinations. It starts with the historical improvement of DNA investigation and its movement in forensics. It then examines the scientific standards and differences between rapid and conventional DNA strategies. Applications of rapid DNA sequencing, including crime scene investigation, distinguishing remains, excusing guiltless people, and understanding cold cases, are identified [1].

2. Historical background of DNA analysis in forensics

The impact of DNA investigation has been enormous on forensic science since it was discovered. This strategy has totally changed the way in which investigators distinguish suspects, absolve innocent individuals, and unravel cases that might otherwise not be illuminated [3]. The procedures of DNA examination have changed significantly in numerous ways over the years, which shows how much innovation and science have altered over time. This segment addresses the history of DNA investigation in forensic science, from a few early strategies that constituted its restriction to finally the issues that drove it to fast DNA sequencing.

2.1 The early days of DNA analysis

DNA was first discovered in the mid-twentieth century as a blueprint of life, yet its application in forensic science did not start until much later. A real breakthrough in the work that Alec Jeffreys completed in 1984 laid the foundation for DNA fingerprinting. Alec Jeffreys developed a technique able to identify unique patterns that exist in the DNA of an individual. This initially emerged from genetic studies but soon acquired its potential for forensic studies [3, 4].

For the first time, DNA evidence was used in a criminal case in 1986. Two young women were murdered in Leicestershire, UK. It failed when it had used conventional methods of investigation, but forensic scientists used DNA profiling to match samples taken from the crime scenes with the suspects' samples. This was the first approach that identified the correct culprit along with freeing the wrongly accused man [1, 2]. It revealed the incredible powers of DNA analysis in bringing justice to mankind and paved its way for acceptance in forensic analysis.

2.2 Restriction fragment length polymorphism (RFLP)

One of the earliest forensic DNA analysis techniques employed is known as Restriction Fragment Length Polymorphism or RFLP. This method was discovered in the 1980s. Under the theory that DNA could be broken down with enzymes called restriction enzymes, each person's DNA varied slightly in size. It is from this variation that forensic experts were able to make a "DNA fingerprint" unique to each person [1–4].

2.3 Advantages of RFLP

1. *High accuracy*: RFLP was very reliable and could differentiate individuals with utmost precision.

2. *Working with larger DNA fragments*: It performed well on high-quality samples that had not broken down.

2.4 Limitations of RFLP

1. *Quality and quantity of sample*: RFLP required sufficient amounts of good quality and intact DNA. Such an amount was generally not feasible in forensic samples obtained during a crime.

2. *Time-consuming process*: The technique was slow, hence taking weeks to yield the results, which made it unsuitable for cases demanding speedy analysis.

3. *Laborious procedures*: RFLP required complex laboratory procedures. This limited its use throughout time-sensitive investigations.

Despite its limitations, RFLP was a pioneering technique that paved the way for modern DNA analysis. It demonstrated the feasibility of using DNA as forensic evidence and paved the way for the development of faster and more efficient techniques [5, 6].

2.5 Polymerase chain reaction (PCR): Revolutionizing DNA analysis

The next big development in DNA analysis came in the form of PCR. Developed by Kary Mullis in the 1980s, PCR is a technique where a small amount of DNA is amplified into millions of copies of a specific DNA segment. This innovation answered most of the challenges with RFLP and very quickly became the backbone of forensic science.

2.5.1 How PCR works

PCR consists of three major steps:

• Denaturation: The DNA is heat denatured to unwind its strands.

• Annealing: Short DNA primers bind to particular target sequences in the DNA.

• Extension: A specific enzyme called Taq polymerase builds new DNA strands by adding nucleotides.

• This is repeated several times, causing the exponential amplification of the target DNA region.

2.5.2 Advantages of PCR

- Works with degraded samples: PCR can amplify even small and degraded DNA samples, making it suitable for forensic investigations.

- Speed: It takes a few hours to complete the whole procedure, much shorter than in the case of RFLP.

- Versatility: PCR can be applied to any type of DNA: nuclear DNA, mitochondrial DNA, and Y-chromosome DNA.

- Only small amounts of DNA are needed, which is a bonus if the evidence is scarce.

2.5.3 Impact of PCR on forensics

It transformed forensic DNA analysis by speeding up the process, increasing accessibility, and making it applicable to a wider variety of samples. It eventually became the method of choice for analyzing biological evidence: blood, bone fragments, hair, and saliva [6].

2.6 The introduction of short tandem repeats (STRs)

PCR became a success, and scientists started to concentrate on particular regions of DNA called Short Tandem Repeats (STRs). STRs are short sequences of DNA that repeat a variable number of times in different individuals [7]. These regions are highly polymorphic, which means they vary greatly between individuals, making them the best for forensic identification [1].

2.7 Advancements in DNA analysis: Toward automation and speed

DNA analysis became more acceptable in forensic science, so it was pursued to automate and facilitate the process. High-throughput DNA sequencing technologies were developed to process large volumes of samples efficiently. Automated systems reduced the likelihood of human error and sped up the analysis, thus making DNA evidence more accessible to law enforcement agencies.

However, despite these developments, traditional DNA analysis techniques had their limitations [8]. Samples were often sent to laboratories where they would be analyzed over a period of days or even weeks. This created an unacceptable delay in the investigation process, especially when time was of the essence—for example, public safety threats or ongoing investigations.

2.8 Limitations of traditional DNA analysis methods

While traditional DNA analysis methods, including RFLP, PCR, and STR analysis, were very reliable, they were not challenge-free:

1. *Time-consuming procedures*: Even the automation of the process of extracting, amplifying, and then analyzing DNA took time.

2. *Dependence on laboratory-based equipment*: DNA analysis required specialized laboratory equipment and a trained personnel member, which barred its accessibility in remote areas or resource-constrained societies.

3. *Preservation problems in samples*: Forensic samples recovered from crime scenes often are degraded or contaminated. Such samples may require considerable time to analyze, thus giving inconclusive results.

4. *Case backlogs*: In most forensic laboratories, DNA testing created a lot of backlogs, making investigations long-winded.

Such issues raised the need for DNA analysis that was quicker, portable, and efficient enough to be used. This set the stage for rapid DNA sequencing [5].

2.9 The paving of the way for rapid DNA sequencing

It was against this background that rapid DNA sequencing technologies were developed. The new technologies aimed at developing systems that would provide accurate DNA results in a fraction of the time taken by the conventional techniques. The foundation of rapid DNA sequencing was through advances in next-generation sequencing (NGS) and third-generation sequencing technologies [9]. Rapid DNA sequencing is a new paradigm for forensic science: it could change the course of investigations by allowing hours rather than days to determine the DNA of an individual. Portable sequencing devices now allow DNA analysis to be carried out at crime scenes themselves, rather than samples needing to be sent to a centralized laboratory [10].

In the following sections, we will see how rapid DNA sequencing builds on the legacy of traditional methods and revolutionizes forensic investigations in unprecedented ways.

3. Development of rapid DNA sequencing

3.1 What is rapid DNA sequencing?

Rapid DNA sequencing involves the advanced process of unraveling the genetic information present within a biological sample in a dramatically shorter time frame, generally a few hours. It is a highly advanced technology compared with earlier DNA analysis techniques that mostly took days or weeks before giving results [1]. These third-generation and next-generation sequencing methods are the primary contributors to this technology since they enable fast and very accurate DNA analysis.

3.2 Key technologies underpinning rapid DNA sequencing

3.2.1 Next-generation sequencing (NGS)

NGS is a revolutionary technology that sequences huge chunks of DNA at once by using parallel processing. In contrast to Sanger sequencing, which reads DNA one fragment at a time, the NGS can sequence the entire genome or particular regions in hours, providing quick and thorough results [3, 4].

3.2.2 Third-generation sequencing

Third-generation sequencing, including nanopore sequencing, reads long DNA strands in real time without fragmentation. DNA is passed through tiny pores in nanopore sequencing, and electrical signals are generated from the DNA sequences. They are portable and user-friendly, making them ideal for on-site forensic investigations [7, 8].

3.3 How does rapid DNA sequencing work?

3.3.1 Sample collection

DNA is taken from biological materials like blood, saliva, or hair at crime scenes, from suspects, or from remains.

3.3.2 Sample preparation

DNA is extracted, broken down if required, and labeled with adapters for sequencing. This is an automated process.

3.3.3 Loading into sequencer

The prepared DNA is put into a sequencing machine. Portable sequencing machines can be used at the site.

3.3.4 DNA sequencing

Devices read DNA bases (A, T, C, and G) and generate a digital sequence. Nanopore sequencing records electrical signals in real time as DNA passes through nanopores.

3.3.5 Data analysis

Digital sequences are analyzed for genetic markers and compared to forensic databases like CODIS to identify individuals or relationships.

3.4 Why is rapid DNA sequencing better?

3.4.1 Speed

Results are obtained within hours rather than days or weeks, which means urgent cases can be decided sooner.

3.4.2 Handles degraded samples

Sensitive technology can process minimal or compromised DNA, which is perfect for forensic evidence.

3.4.3 Portability

Portable devices, such as the Oxford Nanopore MinION, allow DNA to be analyzed on site at crime scenes or in remote locations.

3.4.4 Automation

Automated systems reduce human error and speed up the process, requiring less specialized training.

3.4.5 High accuracy

Advanced technologies such as NGS and nanopore sequencing offer reliable and accurate results.

3.4.6 Cost efficiency

Although devices are costly to purchase, reduced processing times and minimal reliance on the lab make them cost-effective.

3.4.7 Versatility

It analyzes human, microbial, animal, and environmental DNA, which opens up its use beyond forensic applications.

4. Applications of fast DNA sequencing in forensics

- *Crime scene investigation*: The ability to analyze the scene to reduce contamination risk.

- *Remains identification*: Quickly identify victims in disaster or missing persons cases through family DNA.

- *Exoneration*: Accurate results to liberate wrongly accused individuals.

- *Cold case solutions*: To analyze degraded DNA evidence, identifying suspects or new leads.

- *Bioterrorism detection*: Bacterial and viral DNA detection to detect bioterrorism or disease tracking.

- *Paternity testing*: Confirms biological relationships for legal or personal cases.

4.1 Challenges and future prospects

- Costs: Equipment is expensive for some agencies.

- Ethics: Raises privacy concerns about genetic data storage and use.

- Legal issues: Needs standardization for court admissibility.

4.2 Applications in forensic investigations

Rapid DNA sequencing has revolutionized the scope of forensic investigations by way of quick and accurate conclusions, where traditional methods collapse in such situations. Therefore, the ability to interpret DNA within hours has enhanced law enforcement, legal jurisdictions, and disaster response operations' ability to solve critical cases [6, 7]. The major uses of rapid DNA sequencing, their explanations, and detailed examples of its impact appear in the following.

4.3 Crime scene analysis

4.3.1 Suspect and victim identification

Fast DNA sequencing enables forensic teams to match genetic material like blood, hair, or saliva to suspects or victims within hours. It is crucial in high-profile or urgent investigations where immediate answers are necessary. This rapid analysis allows investigators to make quick comparisons of the genetic sequence with forensic databases and thus speed up the case resolution [8, 10].

4.3.2 Real-time decision-making

The versatile gadgets, such as the Oxford Nanopore MinION, can permit DNA investigation on site at any scene. Hence, it becomes conceivable not to take evidence to laboratories for advanced processing, lessening contamination and quickening the investigation pace. It makes possible quick results and makes a difference in taking quick decisions with respect to the detainment of suspects or taking after elective leads, hence highly improving proficiency in cases where critical things are involved [9, 10].

4.3.3 Solving complex cases

With cases involving different numbers of suspects or victims, rapid DNA sequencing offers an opportunity to analyze complex mixtures to unwind each individual's contribution in any given situation. Hence, in a multi-perpetrator theft, one would discover that hereditary samples recovered from a few surfaces may work toward identifying and recognizing among the culprits and in this way render more clarity in complex circumstances [10].

4.4 Identifying unknown remains

Rapid DNA sequencing is utilized to recognize unknown remains when other strategies like fingerprinting or dental records are inaccessible. It provides closure for families by comparing DNA from unidentified remains with reference tests given by relatives in lost people cases, indeed when the skeletal remains are debased [7, 8, 10]. Similarly, the case is for mass calamities, counting those by common catastrophes or terrorist assaults, whereby, due to the speed of DNA sequencing, forensic experts analyze a number of remains collectively and so can indeed distinguish with gross trauma or decomposition in place. It encourages empowering helpful activities in war-torn nations or where human rights have been damaged to also decide the victims and prosecute those responsible on behalf of their families [6].

4.5 Exonerating the innocent

Rapid DNA sequencing has revolutionized the process of absolution, particularly because DNA analysis is no longer slow and costly to access. Organizations such as the Innocence Project proceed to depend on DNA proof to upset wrongful feelings; hence, fast DNA sequencing quickens by analyzing old proof proficiently, and it addresses the issues of backlogged cases inside scientific research facilities, hence centering on examinations including potential wrongful feelings. More so, it prevents miscarriages of justice as clear confirmation is set amid an initial organization of examination [9]. It decreases reliance on circumstantial or questionable eyewitness accounts.

4.6 Cold case resolutions

Rapid DNA sequencing helps significantly in cold cases that involved biological evidence collected when such techniques as modern DNA techniques were not available [3]. The technology can analyze degraded evidence and has led to breakthroughs, such as those witnessed in the Golden State Killer case. By making genealogical comparisons, it creates new leads by familial searching, thereby rapidly narrowing the list of possible suspects [5]. For the victims' families, rapid DNA sequencing gives them hope and a possibility of closure with regard to longstanding mysteries.

4.7 Mass disaster victim identification

DNA sequencing that can be conducted quickly became necessary in the management of large-scale casualty incidents when it comes to identification events. It would enable multiple samples to be processed as a batch in forensic examination teams and thus accelerate efforts in incidents such as plane crashes and earthquakes; hence, there is emotional reduction on the families over the loved ones. Disaster response plans more and more contain provisions for rapid DNA sequencing, thereby equipping forensic teams for efficient identification [5]. Furthermore, in cross-border incidents, the technology assists in cooperation by giving standard results that can be easily shared across borders [1].

4.8 Border security and immigration

Rapid DNA sequencing is revolutionizing border security and immigration processes through a guaranteed way of establishing familial relations to prevent fraud. This is helpful in that the claim of blood relationship should be authentic in refugee situations, as the separation of children from parents has to be prevented. In addition, the technology prevents human trafficking, for false claims of blood relationships may be found to determine efficient intervention. Through speeding up processing time, the use of rapid DNA sequencing allows legitimate immigration cases to be resolved in time. It also boosts border security through identity verification and detection of forged documents to further strengthen the protection layers of immigration systems [6, 7].

5. Case studies: Real-life applications of rapid DNA sequencing

The transformative capability of rapid DNA sequencing makes sense best through real-case examples. This section considers one very interesting case history in which rapid DNA sequencing was crucial to solving the murder mystery of decades past.

This case shows that this advanced technology has turned the world of forensic science upside down and has indeed contributed to justice and humanity [4].

5.1 Case: Solving a decades-old murder

5.1.1 Background

In the 1980s, a young woman was killed inside her apartment in an atrocious manner. In the investigations, all their best efforts were in vain; it went cold. Among the evidence recovered at the crime scene was some biological material, for instance, a bloodstain found on the clothing of the victim and a strand of hair that was seen on the body. But since RFLP is used, high-quality samples containing DNA must be huge and of an enormous size. Unfortunately, the recovered samples were small and partially degraded and thus could not be used with traditional methods.

For decades, the victim's family sought justice, but the case remained unsolved due to technological limitations [5]. It was only when recent advancements in rapid DNA sequencing allowed investigators to revisit the evidence that they were finally able to uncover the truth.

5.2 Solving cold cases using rapid DNA sequencing

It has turned out to be very helpful in solving cold cases through the re-examination of degraded evidence. For example, investigators applied NGS to extract full DNA profiles from biological samples decades old—a bloodstain and a hair sample. A DNA profile matched the suspect in a national database in hours, with a record of unrelated crimes [3]. Further analysis of the cigarette butt from the crime scene confirmed the same DNA profile, which was an added strength to the evidence. The suspect was caught, confessed, and convicted. This brought long-awaited justice to the victim's family. The case opened doors for revisiting unsolved cases by using advanced forensic tools, inspiring renewed investigations worldwide [4].

5.3 Outcome and impact

Rapid DNA sequencing improved the identification of victims within mass disasters so much that families were able to close their cases within weeks rather than months or years. This success created a worldwide precedent and set disaster response plans with the integration of rapid DNA technology into these plans. Moreover, there was a high need for portable devices in such hard environments. Psychological effects were minimized, and public trust in governments and humanitarian organizations increased [5]. These cases illustrate the applicability, effectiveness, and accuracy of fast DNA sequencing. It, in its critical role, was decisive for solving crimes, ensuring justice, and filling humanitarian needs.

The following case studies serve as proof of the wide reach and impact of accelerated DNA sequencing in forensic practice. Because it allows quick yet highly reliable DNA profiling, it has changed all those previous ways of processing the crime scene and, on other occasions, doing identifications of victims, not just in solving those so-called cold cases but in dealing with what sometimes results from mass disaster catastrophes. This technology will continue to expand its applications and impact the more it evolves, securing its place as a primary tool in forensic science [3].

Technique	Time required	Accuracy	Advantages	Limitations
RFLP	Weeks	High	Reliable for large samples	Time-consuming, needs high-quality DNA
PCR	Hours	High	Works with degraded samples	Requires specific primers, false positives
STR	Hours	Very high	Efficient for identification	Depends on sample quality
Rapid DNA	Hours (real-time)	Very high	Quick, portable, on-site use	Expensive, complex data analysis

Table 1.
DNA analysis technology comparison.

5.4 Challenges and limitations of rapid DNA sequencing

Although a very useful tool for rapid DNA sequencing, the technology has some challenges. It is expensive to procure, and the cost of equipment and materials is relatively high, which makes it hard for smaller labs, especially in developing areas, to afford [7]. This limits its use to important cases. To make it more affordable, advancements in technology and support from the government or private sector are needed. Also, big data of DNA is really hard to analyze and can only be done by experts; without a standard method, results vary. Using such tools as AI and even more training for experts will help to increase accuracy and the speed of understanding the data (**Table 1**).

6. Contamination risks, legal hurdles, and ethical concerns

6.1 Contamination risks

Biological samples may be contaminated with factors from the environment or handling in the laboratory, and this can lead to misleading results. Strict protocols of handling, storage, and equipment maintenance, along with quality control measures, reduce these risks [8].

6.2 Legal hurdles

It should be compatible with strict legal standards. Rapid DNA sequencing may trigger a legal challenge because many feel that the results produced by this technique are unreliable in comparison to the traditional approach. Proper documentation and custody of the DNA samples are indispensable for avoiding legal issues [8].

6.3 Ethical concerns

DNA data contains sensitive information, which raises issues about privacy and consent. Misuse can also be found in the form of using DNA databases for surveillance or discrimination [5].

7. Legal and ethical considerations for rapid DNA sequencing

7.1 Privacy considerations

DNA holds highly sensitive data at the individual level; thus, it can result in extreme implications if accessed and utilized without authorization or perniciously [9]. Forensic DNA databases require adequate cybersecurity affirmation to be assured to guarantee security. Risks prevail in re-identification in the event that DNA profiles are de-anonymized.

7.2 Informed consent

Collecting DNA without informed consent is unethical and legally questionable. Communication must be straightforward so that individuals know what their DNA will be used for [5]. However, where a criminal investigation is required, for example, a balance must be struck in the individual's rights to public safety.

7.3 Bias and discrimination

This means that there is the risk of using DNA databases in the unfair targeting of particular groups, hence discrimination. Safeguards for the prevention of misuse beyond forensic purposes are necessary [10].

7.4 Regulation of rapid DNA technologies

There's a need to establish clear rules on the application of rapid DNA sequencing in forensic examinations with a view to precision, approval, and court suitability. Independent oversight and regular audits can be useful to guarantee that the innovation is utilized ethically and responsibly [9].

8. Future directions and innovations in rapid DNA sequencing

8.1 Portable DNA sequencers

Handheld DNA sequencers are currently being created that can specifically analyze at a crime scene. They will speed up examinations and avoid defilement. They can also be utilized in calamity reaction and border security to rapidly distinguish victims and confirm family relationships in real time [5].

8.2 AI integration

AI can prepare DNA information faster and more precisely, with fewer mistakes. Prescient AI instruments might also be able to tell physical characteristics or ancestry from DNA, which might open up modern leads for an examination [5].

8.3 Improved accessibility

With advancing technology, it will decrease the cost of DNA sequencing, hence indeed empowering littler labs and less progressed nations to perform these arrangements [9]. This would subsequently increase the effect of fast DNA sequencing around the world in tackling violations and understanding helpful issues.

8.4 Predictive capabilities

Future progress may even be able to allow forensic researchers to predict physical features based on DNA, counting eye color and stature. The study of predicting well-being or behavioral characteristics may have measurable applications, but such efforts raise extreme ethical concerns [6].

8.5 Integration with other forensic tools

Rapid DNA sequencing can work in synergy with other forensic strategies, like unique finger impression filtering or facial recognition. For this reason, investigators have to be able to come up with more well-articulated cases and ideally appreciate a smoother criminal justice process [6, 7].

9. Conclusion

Rapid DNA sequencing has had a huge effect on current forensic examinations, with rapid acceleration in the speed, exactness, and proficiency of DNA investigation. The innovation is demonstrated to be valuable to break crimes, excuse the innocent, and establish identities in timely situations, including mass disasters or ongoing crimes. Its ability to work on smaller, corrupted tests rapidly and donate real-time data has revolutionized workflows in scientific research facilities. In addition to the challenges of having a tall, fetched, complex interpretation of data and issues regarding morals, the stable development of rapid DNA sequencing innovation is promising for future applications in forensic science. Further enhancements along the lines of availabilities, the utilization of versatile sequencing gadgets, and AI integration into these gadgets will alter the face of criminal equity all over the world. As the legal and moral system surrounding its use proceeds to advance, rapid DNA sequencing will remain a critical element within the conveyance of equity, improvement of forensic investigation, and accountability.

Acknowledgements

I extend heartfelt gratitude to Muhammad Rehan for his insightful guidance and support, which significantly enriched this book chapter.

The author acknowledges the usage of Chat GPT for language polishing of the manuscript.

Nomenclature

DNA	deoxyribonucleic acid
PCR	polymerase chain reaction
STR	short tandem repeat
RFLP	restriction fragment length polymorphism
NGS	next-generation sequencing
AI	artificial intelligence

Author details

Asma Jan Muhammad
Institute of Molecular Biology and Biotechnology, Bahauddin Zakariya University,
Multan, Pakistan

*Address all correspondence to: asmajanmohammad@gmail.com

IntechOpen

References

[1] Murphy E. Forensic DNA typing. Annual Review of Criminology. 2018;**1**(1):497-515. DOI: 10.1146/annurev-criminol-032317-092127

[2] Singh A, Rawtani D. DNA sequencing and rapid DNA tests. In: Modern Forensic Tools and Devices: Trends in Criminal Investigation. Hoboken, NJ: John Wiley & Sons, Inc.; 2023. pp. 225-264. DOI: 10.1002/9781119763406.ch10

[3] Alketbi SK. Emerging technologies in forensic DNA analysis. Perspectives in Legal and Forensic Sciences. 2024;**1**(1):1-24. DOI: 10.70322/plfs.2024.10007

[4] Erlich H, Calloway C, Lee SB. Recent developments in forensic DNA technology. In: Silent Witness: Forensic DNA Analysis in Criminal Investigations and Humanitarian Disasters. Springer; 2020. pp. 105-127. Available from: https://www.researchgate.net/publication/349087715

[5] Alketbi SK. The role of DNA in forensic science: A comprehensive review. International Journal of Science and Research Archive. 2023;**9**(02):814-829. DOI: 10.30574/ijsra.2023.9.2.0624

[6] Chong KW, Thong Z, Syn CK. Recent trends and developments in forensic DNA extraction. Wiley Interdisciplinary Reviews: Forensic Science. 2021;**3**(2):e1395. DOI: 10.1002/wfs2.1395

[7] Dash HR, Elkins KM, Al-Snan NR, Dash HR. Advancements in forensic DNA analysis. Singapore: Springer Nature; 2023. DOI: 10.1007/978-981-99-6195-5

[8] Bhosale M, Seth R, Nanhe B. Forensic DNA biomarkers: Advancements and applications in criminal investigations. Biochemical & Cellular Archives. 2023;**23**(2):1297-1303. DOI: 10.51470/bca.2023.23.2.1297

[9] Allwood JS, Fierer N, Dunn RR. The future of environmental DNA in forensic science. Applied and Environmental Microbiology. 2020;**86**(2):e01504-e01519. DOI: 10.1128/AEM.01504-19

[10] Butler JM. The future of forensic DNA analysis. Philosophical Transactions of the Royal Society B: Biological Sciences. 2015;**370**(1674):20140252. DOI: 10.1098/rstb.2014.0252

Chapter 3

Application of Energy-Dispersive X-Ray Fluorescence Spectrometry for Examination of Foreign Bodies in Forensic Practice

Sella Takei, Hiroshi Kinoshita and Takehiko Murase

Abstract

We review here the application of energy-dispersive X-ray fluorescence spectrometry (EDX), a simultaneous and non-destructive technique for multi-element analysis that is applicable to determine the elemental composition of a sample without any special preparation. EDX is widely used for compositional analyses of materials such as metal, cement, glass, petrochemicals and geological samples in industrial and scientific fields. However, the application of EDX to forensic practice has been limited to date. The present paper discusses the application of EDX to the examination of foreign bodies in forensic practice. As EDX provide various information, it is useful for the identification of foreign body, and further application in this field would be expected.

Keywords: energy-dispersive X-ray fluorescence spectrometry (EDX), foreign body, forensic practice, element analysis, forensic pathology

1. Introduction

Various examinations are routinely performed in daily forensic practice. Postmortem computed tomography (PMCT), blood typing, biochemistry, histopathology, radiology, and alcohol, drug and toxicological testing are performed alongside autopsies. Diatom tests may also be performed in cases when drowning is suspected, and DNA analysis may be performed if necessary to confirm the identity of the deceased [1]. When foreign bodies are found during inspections, a detailed visual examination is usually performed first. If the origin of the foreign bodies requires investigation, more detailed examinations are required.

Identification of foreign bodies is primarily performed according to morphological characteristics. However, this information alone may not provide enough evidence, and the results of chemical analysis can be helpful in making a conclusive identification [2].

Morphological examinations of foreign bodies may involve not only observation with the naked eye, but also observations using a stereomicroscope, optical microscope, and electron microscope. However, using an optical microscope or electron microscope requires sample preparation, which in turn involves some degree of destruction of the sample. Observation is first performed using a stereomicroscope in most cases, followed by element analysis using a non-destructive method like energy-dispersive X-ray fluorescence spectrometry (EDX). If there is a possibility that the foreign matter is organic, the use of Fourier-transform infrared spectroscopy (FT-IR) is also considered [3]. While examination of foreign bodies is not required particularly often in daily forensic practice, particularly in forensic autopsies, a certain demand remains. When a foreign body is found during medical practice in a hospital, consistent procedures to conduct such examinations are typically lacking and the doctor in charge is left wondering how to request them. For this reason, consultations and measurements are often requested to forensic laboratories. We provide herein an overview of the role of EDX in foreign body examinations from the perspective of forensic medicine.

2. EDX

EDX is an analytical method for the qualitative and quantitative analysis of constituent elements. The method is non-destructive, allows simultaneous analysis of multiple elements [3–8], and measurements can be performed easily without special sample pretreatment. EDX is widely used for quality control in the fields of industry and environmental analysis, such as analyses of metal impurities, cement components, petrochemicals, and testing for environmental pollutants. Use in the analysis of debris, soil, and dental prostheses or dental materials has also been reported in the field of forensic science [9–12]. However, descriptions of applications to biological samples remain relatively scarce [13–17]. An EDX device coupled with scanning electron microscopy (SEM/EDX) [9, 13, 18–24] or X-ray scanning analytical microscopy (XSAM) [25] is capable of performing elemental analysis as well as allowing morphological observation. SEM/EDX is known as an analytical electron microscope and is widely used in the examination of microscopic objects.

3. Principles of EDX measurements

EDX is a method to analyze constituent elements and compositional ratios of substances based on the energy and intensity of fluorescent X-rays generated when the sample is irradiated with X-rays. The energy of fluorescent X-rays is determined for each element, and the intensity of the fluorescent X-rays is related to the amount of an element contained in the sample.

When an atom receives an X-ray, the energy of the X-ray is transferred to the atom. If the energy of radiation is sufficiently large, electrons in the inner shells are ejected and create vacancies (excited state). This condition is unstable, and electrons from the outer shells transfer to the inner vacancies, returning the unstable atom to a stable condition (ground state). Between these two states, the excess energy is released as a characteristic X-ray that is specific to each element (**Figure 1**) [4–8, 26]. EDX measures the intensity and energy of these characteristic X-rays (**Figure 2**).

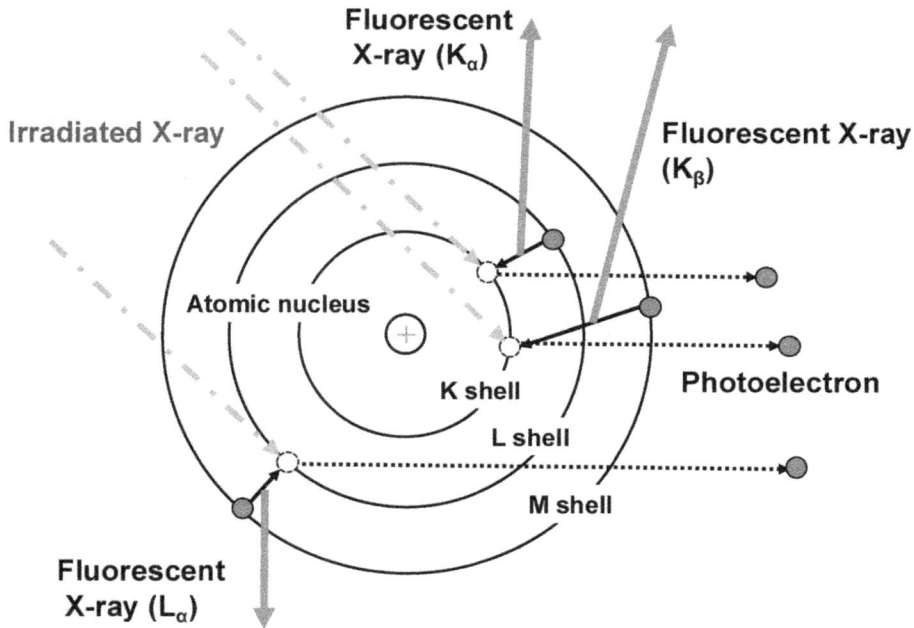

Figure 1.
Mechanism of fluorescent X-ray generation. (Cited from [26], with permission).

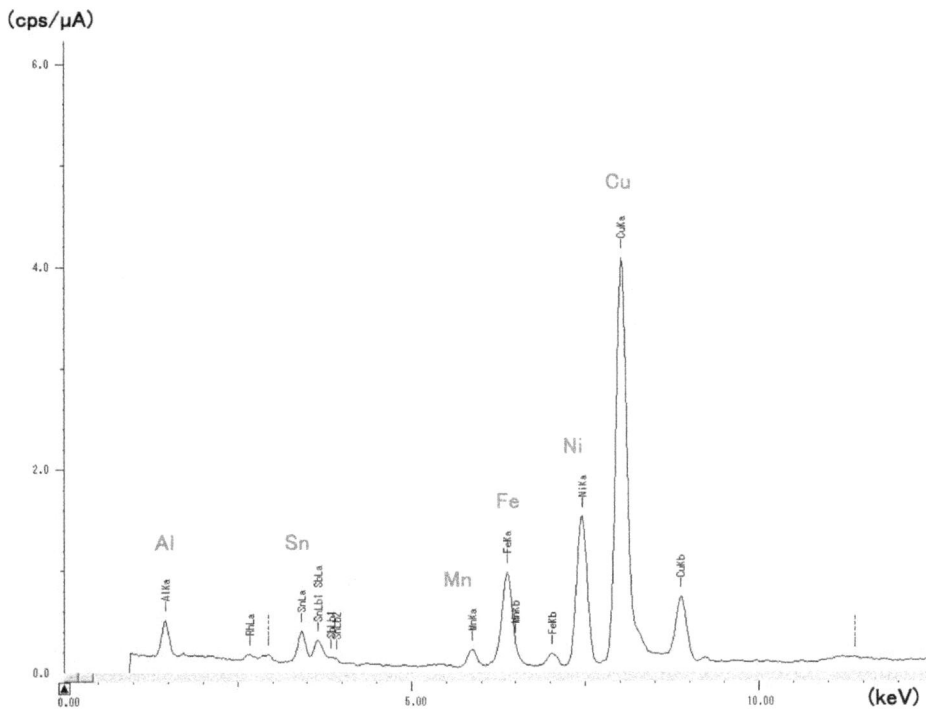

Figure 2.
Representative EDX spectrum shows characteristic peaks of each element.

Elements are thus identified from the energy, while the X-ray intensity, shown as peak height, is used for quantitative analysis [4–8, 26].

X-rays have a highly penetrative property, allowing application to non-destructive analysis of solids, liquids, and powders [4–8, 26]. The characteristic X-rays emitted in a vacuum are not attenuated by air, enabling measurements with low baseline and high sensitivity. However, as measurements of liquid and powder samples cannot be performed under vacuum conditions, we have to consider other measurement methods. For example, measurement of a liquid sample could be applied not only to the sample directly but also to the liquid dripped within a paraffin circle on filter paper and dried before EDX measurement [5, 8, 17, 27].

4. Benefits of using EDX for examination of foreign bodies

As mentioned earlier, non-destructive testing can be conducted for samples in various forms, such as solids, powders, and liquids, using simple procedures. This is quite useful when qualitative elemental analysis is required [4–8, 26].

5. Applications of EDX for examination of foreign bodies

We present some examples, focusing on reported applications and our results so far.

5.1 Estimation of equipment used

5.1.1 Bullet analysis (fragmentation/debris)

(Case study) A minute metallic foreign body was found at autopsy in a wound on the back of the head of a male who had committed suicide with a handgun. Lead and antimony were detected from the EDX of the foreign body. As these elements are typically the main components of bullets, the foreign body was considered to be part of a fragmented bullet. Based on the autopsy findings, the direct cause of death was concluded to be brain contusion caused by the passage of the bullet [28]. In addition, lead was also successfully detected in the skin surrounding the area through which the bullet had passed (gunshot wound) [29]. The results of EDX and the form and shape of the wound provided useful information.

5.1.2 Analysis of deposits around a lesion

Cases are sometimes encountered in which a bullet has passed through the body (penetrating gunshot wounds). The direction of entry of the bullet provides important information as to the nature of the crime and is usually judged from the morphological characteristics of the wound [30]. This allows for accurate judgment in most cases, but judgment is difficult in some cases. Chemical identification methods using atomic absorption spectrometry or inductively coupled plasma-atomic emission spectrometry (ICP-AES) have been reported to allow identification of the entrance wound based on the amount of lead around the wound [31, 32], but pretreatment dissolving the tissue is required with such methods. When EDX was used to directly measure lead levels in tissue samples fixed in formalin, the entrance and exit wounds could be clearly distinguished [33]. In that case, EDX analysis of foreign substances around the wound provided useful information as to the nature of the crime.

5.1.3 Identification of equipment or material

In some cases, parts of the equipment or material involved in the death remain after the injury has been caused. (Case study) A small fragment was found in a wound in the back of the head of a man found dead on a riverbank with stones lying around nearby. EDX analysis of fragments removed during autopsy confirmed that those fragments originated from a stone [34]. The instrument or material (e.g., iron pipe, hammer, or wood) itself does not remain in place in most cases, but fragments or blade components can reportedly be detected by EDX [35, 36], and the results of analysis are thus useful for estimating what was involved in a person's death.

5.2 Examinations for foreign bodies in the body

5.2.1 Identification of iodine

(Case study) An elderly man died after being involved in a car accident while walking along the road. PMCT performed before autopsy revealed granular high-density areas not associated with hemorrhage, mainly at the base of the brain (**Figure 3a**). Similar high-density areas were also seen in the spinal canal. The autopsy revealed hemopneumothorax with multiple bilateral rib fractures, lung and liver contusions, and pelvic fractures. The cause of death was concluded to be traumatic shock due to severe trauma to the trunk. Autopsy of the brain revealed mild traumatic subarachnoid hemorrhage and yellow granules the size of rice grains attached to the base of the brain (**Figure 3b**). EDX of these granules revealed iodine (**Figure 4**). These findings were thus thought to represent remnants of iophendylate, an oil-based contrast agent that was used in spinal cord imaging until the early 1980s. Although remnant contrast agent was not considered directly related to the cause of death, EDX provided evidence that the patient had a medical history of procedures involving contrast agents [37].

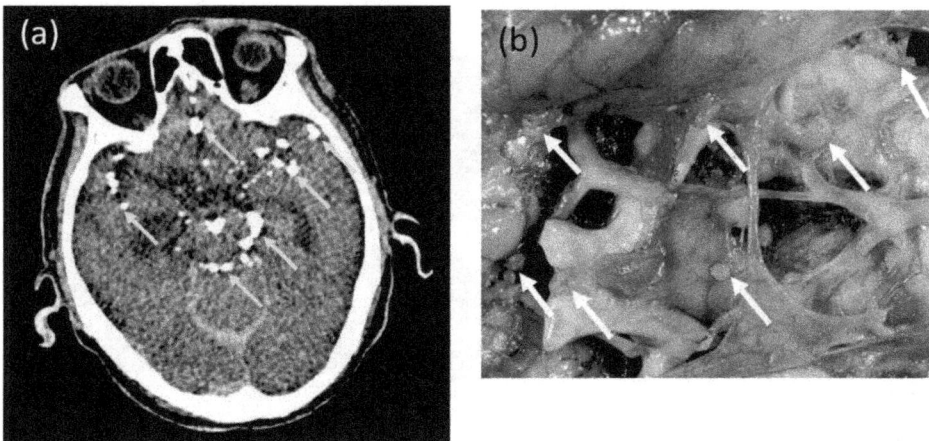

Figure 3.
(a) High-density area in the skull (yellow arrow). (b) Yellow granules at the base of the brain (white arrow). (Cited from [37], with permission).

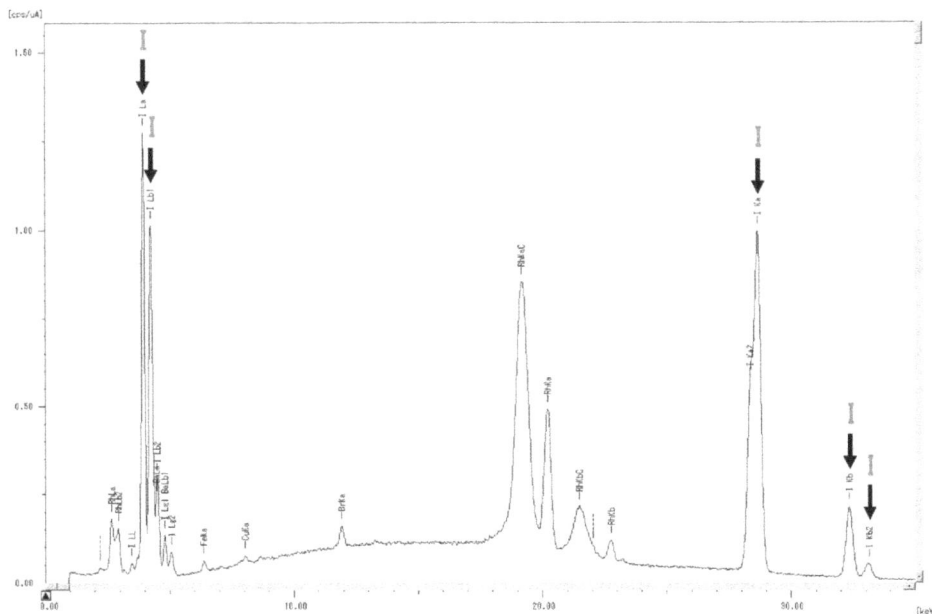

Figure 4.
EDX spectrum of the yellow granule. (Cited from [37], with permission).

5.3 Examination of gastrointestinal contents

5.3.1 Remnants of barium contrast media

(Case study) A man was found dead in a river. PMCT performed before autopsy confirmed a high-density area with artifacts in the ascending colon (**Figure 5a**). The autopsy also revealed a white stone, approximately 1.5 cm in diameter, at the same site (**Figure 5b**). EDX revealed barium as the main component of the stone (**Figure 6**). Barium is primarily used as a contrast agent in examinations of the gastrointestinal tract. Barium is naturally excreted after the examination in most cases but can lead to

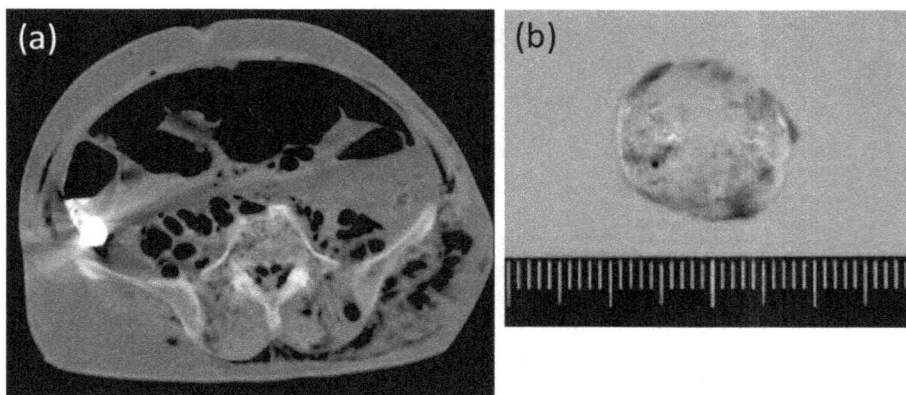

Figure 5.
(a) High-density area in the ascending colon. (b) White stone matching the location identified on imaging. (Cited from [38], with permission).

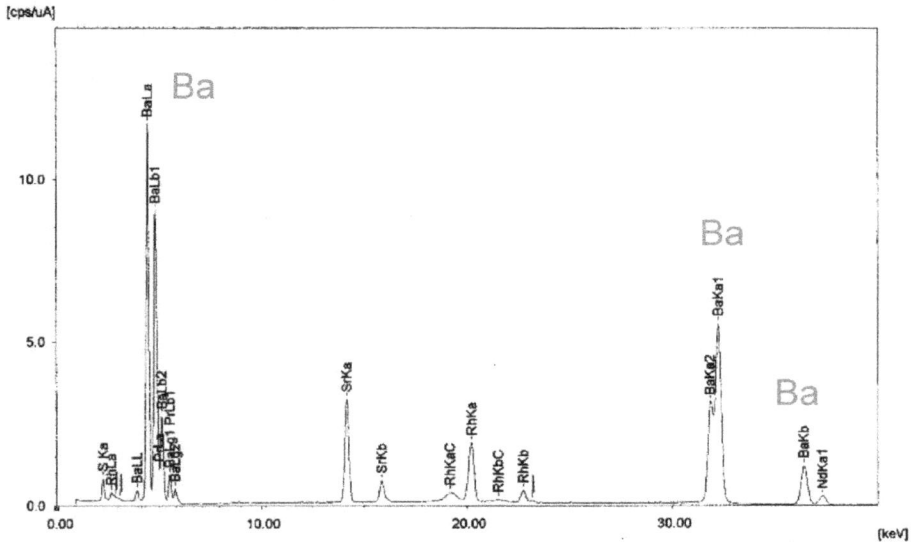

Figure 6.
EDX spectrum of the white stone. (Cited from [38], with permission).

complications such as intestinal obstruction or colonic perforation in a small number of cases. The residual barium contrast agent indicated that the patient had undergone gastrointestinal contrast examination before death. However, the dates of such examinations are generally difficult to identify in autopsy cases [38].

5.3.2 Confirmation of fishbone

When foreign bodies are obtained from surgical specimens, clear identification is important in pathological evaluations [39]. (Case study) A black, elongated foreign body was removed from the surgical site of a woman in her 80s who had undergone surgery for colon perforation. EDX revealed that the substance contained high proportions of calcium and phosphorus. This result made it unlikely that the body was an organic material such as plastic. Under histological examination, the foreign object was revealed to morphologically resemble bone. Based on the size and test results, the foreign body was concluded to be a fish bone [40].

5.3.3 Evidence of ingestion of poisonous substances

Qualitative and quantitative analyses for the involvement of poisons or toxic chemicals are performed in cases where poisoning is suspected, and stomach contents may be examined in addition to blood and urine. EDX is considered useful in screening for aluminum, phosphorus, sulfur, chromium, arsenic, bromine, cadmium, mercury, thallium, and lead [4]. There have been reports in which EDX was applied to cases of fatal ingestion of mercury [41] and the detection of arsenic in stomach contents [42, 43].

EDX analysis only provides information on elemental constituents, not on chemical compositions or structures. Organophosphate and carbamate pesticides contain phosphorus and sulfur in their chemical structures, respectively, and examinations for these elements in high concentrations may thus be used as a screening test [4]. When relatively high peaks for phosphorus or sulfur are detected from samples of stomach contents, the possibility of organophosphate or carbamate ingestion should be considered [44, 45]. In addition, cases have been reported in which silicon peaks were detected in stomach contents from products to which silicic acid or other substances have been added [45].

5.3.4 Screening for drug overdose

Bromovalerylurea is used as a hypnotic and contains bromine, allowing screening tests using bromine as an indicator [46, 47].

Detection of additives can be useful in cases of drug overdose [48]. (Case study) A man was found dead in his house. He had been prescribed various hypnotics and psychotropic drugs, and many empty packages were also found inside the room where his body was discovered. EDX examination of the stomach contents detected titanium, silicon, and magnesium. Subsequent toxicological examinations also identified many psychotropic drugs at relatively high concentrations. Magnesium stearate is added to psychotropic drugs as a lubricant to ensure fluidity. Silicic anhydride is used as a flow agent and titanium oxide and talc (hydrated magnesium silicate) are added to tablets to block light and prevent the drug from sticking [49]. EDX examination of the stomach contents is thus useful when tablets containing these elements are ingested, particularly in cases of overdose [50].

5.4 Examination of dental prosthesis

When skeletal remains are discovered, clues for identification must be gathered. Information about the teeth, including dentures and dental prostheses, often provides strong clues for identification [39]. Any information on the specific components of dentures or prostheses thus becomes even more useful. Analysis of the components of metal crowns by EDX can reveal the types of alloys present, such as gold-silver-palladium alloy and nickel-palladium alloy, representing useful information for personal identification [51, 52]. In addition, when analyzing foreign objects found in food, EDX is highly useful for detecting foreign objects, which are often fragments of dental materials [3].

6. Summary and future prospects

We have summarized the utility of EDX analysis for the investigation of foreign bodies in daily forensic practice, focusing on previous reports. Detailed examination of foreign bodies is required in many situations, providing a wide array of information such as a basis for inferring the condition of an individual or their medical history during life. We hope that this method will continue to be more actively applied in practice. Further case studies and accumulation of results are required with regard to the application of EDX analysis in daily practice.

Acknowledgements

We wish to thank Dr. Naoko Tanaka and Ms. Ayaka Yasumoto-Takakura for their technical support.

Application of Energy-Dispersive X-Ray Fluorescence Spectrometry for Examination of Foreign...
DOI: http://dx.doi.org/10.5772/intechopen.1009220

The authors thank FORTE Science Communications (https://www.forte-science.co.jp/) for English language editing.

This work was partially supported by JSPS KAKENHI Grant-in-Aid for Young Scientists (Start-up) Number 22K21173 and Grant-in-Aid for Scientific Research (C) Number 21K10524.

Conflict of interest

The authors declare no conflict of interest.

Author details

Sella Takei[1], Hiroshi Kinoshita[2]* and Takehiko Murase[1]

1 Department of Forensic Medicine, Faculty of Medicine, Kagawa University, Kita, Kagawa, Japan

2 National Research Institute of Police Science, Kashiwa, Chiba, Japan

*Address all correspondence to: kinochin7587@gmail.com

IntechOpen

References

[1] Ikematsu K, Abe Y, Shinba Y, Yamashita H, Murase T. Introduction of testing in forensic practice. Journal of Japanese Society of Laboratory Medicine. 2024;**72**:607-611

[2] Jackson ARW, Jackson JM. Forensic Science. Essex: Pearson Education; 2004

[3] Ito S, Ikeda Y, Kawakami T, Saito T. Analysis of foreign substances found in food. Journal of Dental Health. 2015;**65**:403-409

[4] Namera A, Namiki K. New analytical techniques for determination of toxins -3- X-ray fluorescence spectroscopy. Chūdoku Kenkyū. 2000;**13**:91-97

[5] Kawai J. Expert Series for Analytical Chemistry Instrumentation Analysis, X-ray Fluorescence analysis. Vol. 6. Tokyo: Kyoritsu Shuppan; 2012

[6] Marguí E, Grieken RV. X-Ray Fluorescence Spectrometry and Related Techniques. New York: Momentum Press; 2013

[7] Stuart BH. Forensic Analytical Techniques. West Sussex: John Wiley & Sons Ltd; 2013

[8] Nakai I, editor. Practice of Fluorescent X-Ray Analysis. 2nd ed. Tokyo: Asakura-Syoten; 2016

[9] Merelli V, Caccia G, Mazzarelli D, Franceschetti L, Paciello O, Bonizzoni L, et al. Skin surface debris as an archive of environmental traces: An investigation through the naked eye, episcopic microscope, ED-XRF, and SEM-EDX. International Journal of Legal Medicine. 2024;**138**:123-137. DOI: 10.1007/s00414-023-03021-1

[10] Gordon SC, Daley TD. Foreign body gingivitis. Identification of the foreign material by energy-dispersive x-ray microanalysis. Oral Surgery, Oral Medicine, Oral Pathology, Oral Radiology, and Endodontics. 1997;**83**:571-576. DOI: 10.1016/s1079-2104(97)90122-0

[11] Aboshi H, Takahashi T, Komura T. Component analysis of dental porcelain for assisting dental identification. The Journal of Forensic Odonto-Stomatology. 2006;**24**:36-41

[12] Uitdehaag S, Wiarda W, Donders T, Kuiper I. Forensic comparison of soil samples using nondestructive elemental analysis. Journal of Forensic Sciences. 2017;**62**:861-868. DOI: 10.1111/1566-4029.13313

[13] Seta S, Sato H, Mamba K, Sudo T. Application of the energy-dispersive X-ray microanalyzer equipped with the scanning electron microscope to the criminal identification of body fluid stains. Nihon Hōigaku Zasshi. 1976;**30**:371-379

[14] Rastegar F, Maier EA, Heimburger R, Christophe C, Ruch C, Leroy MJF. Simultaneous determination of trace elements in serum by energy-dispersive X-ray fluorescence spectrometry. Clinical Chemistry. 1984;**30**:1300-1303

[15] Börjesson J, Isaksson M, Mattsson S. X-ray fluorescence analysis in medical sciences: A review. Acta Diabetologica. 2003;**40**:S39-S44. DOI: 10.1007/s00592-003-0024-z

[16] Uo M, Wada T, Sugiyama T. Application of X-ray fluorescence analysis (XRF) to dental and medical specimens. Japanese Dental Science

Review. 2015;**51**:2-9. DOI: 10.1016/j.jdsr.2014.07.001

[17] Tanaka H, Nakajima M, Fujisawa M, Kasamaki M, Hori Y, Yoshikawa H, et al. Rapid determination of total bromide in human serum using an energy-dispersive X-ray spectrometer. Biological & Pharmaceutical Bulletin. 2003;**26**:457-461. DOI: 10.1248/bpb.26.457

[18] DiMaio VJM, Dana SE, Taylor WE, Ondrusek J. Use of scanning electron microscopy and energy dispersive X-ray analysis (SEM-EDXA) in identification of foreign material on bullets. Journal of Forensic Sciences. 1987;**32**:38-47

[19] Zadora G, Brożek-Mucha Z. SEM-EDX—A useful tool for forensic examinations. Materials Chemistry and Physics. 2003;**81**:345-348

[20] Cengiz S, Karaca AC, Çakir İ, Üner HB, Sevindik A. SEM-EDS analysis and discrimination of forensic soil. Forensic Science International. 2004;**141**:33-37. DOI: 10.1016/j.jigo.2014.10.023

[21] Kinoshita H, Nishiguchi M, Ouchi H, Minami T, Kubota A, Utsumi T, et al. The application of variable-pressure scanning electron microscope with energy dispersive X-ray microanalyzer to the diagnosis of electrocution: A case report. Legal Medicine. 2004;**6**:55-60. DOI: 10.1016/j.legalmed.2003.08.006

[22] Bush MA, Raymond RG, Norrlander AL, Bush PJ. Analytical survey of restorative resins by SEM/EDX and XRF: Databases for forensic purposes. Journal of Forensic Sciences. 2008;**53**:419-425. DOI: 10.1111/j.1556-4029.2007.00654.x

[23] Gentile G, Andreola S, Bailo P, Battistini A, Boracchi M, Tambuzzi S, et al. A brief review of scanning electron microscopy with energy-dispersive X-ray use in forensic medicine. The American Journal of Forensic Medicine and Pathology. 2020;**41**:280-286. DOI: 10.1097/PAF.0000000000000609

[24] Matsui K, Ueno T, Takahashi M, Nagai T, Suzuki K, Kinoshita H. A study of asbestos bodies using scanning electron microscopy with energy dispersive X-ray microanalysis (SEM-EDX). Current Study Environmental Medicine Science. 2009;**2**:3-5

[25] Uo M, Watari F. Rapid analysis of metallic dental restorations using X-ray scanning analytical microscopy. Dental Materials. 2004;**20**:611-615. DOI: 10.1016/j.dental.2003.08.002

[26] Tanaka N, Kinoshita H. Application of energy dispersive X-ray fluorescent spectrometry (EDX) in the field of forensic pathology. Forensic Pathology. 2018;**24**:131-137

[27] Tanaka N, Kinoshita H, Jamal M, Takakura A, Kumihashi M, Miyatake N, et al. Detection of chlorine and bromine in free liquid from the sphenoid sinus as an indicator of seawater drowning. Legal Medicine. 2015;**17**:299-303. DOI: 10.1016/j.legalmed.2015.08.005

[28] Kinoshita H, Nishiguchi M, Kasuda S, Matsui K, Ouchi H, Minami T, et al. Application of energy dispersive X-ray fluorescent spectroscopy (EDXRF) in the field of forensic medicine: Identification of lethal weapon. Medical Biology. 2008;**152**:108-111

[29] Takahashi M, Kinoshita H, Nishiguchi M, Nishio H. Detection of metallic elements from paraffin-embedded tissue blocks by energy dispersive X-ray fluorescence spectrometry. Legal Medicine. 2010;**12**:102-103. DOI: 10.1016/j.legalmed.2009.12.003

[30] Di Maio VJM. Gunshot Wounds. Practical Aspects of Firearms, Ballistics, and Forensic Techniques. 2nd ed. Boca Raton, London: CRC Press; 1999

[31] Otsuji M, Rohwer J, Oehmichen M, Oshima T. Inorganic lead concentration analysis at the gunshot wounds for differentiation of entrance from exit hole. Acta Criminologiae et Medicinae Lagalis Japonica. 1998;**64**:213-218

[32] Wunnapuk K, Durongkadech P, Minami T, Ruangyuttikarn W, Tohno S, Vichairat K, et al. Differences in the element contents between gunshot entry wounds with full-jacketed bullet and lead bullet. Biological Trace Element Research. 2007;**120**:74-81. DOI: 10.1007/s12011-007-8014-6

[33] Tanaka N, Kinoshita H, Takakura A, Jamal M, Ito A, Kumihashi M, et al. Distinction between entrance and exit wounds by energy dispersive X-ray fluorescence spectrometry. Legal Medicine. 2016;**22**:5-8. DOI: 10.1016/j.legalmed.2016.07.003

[34] Kinoshita H, Tanaka N, Jamal M, Yamashita T, Kimura S. Identification of foreign body using energy-dispersive X-ray fluorescence spectrometry. New Bulletin of Medical Science. 2020;**4**(3):3-6

[35] Zhu Y, Tao X, Li Z, Chen L, Zhou W. A study on identification of the blunt lethal objects of wood, iron, brick and stone in homicide by SEM and EDAX. Nihon Hōigaku Zasshi. 1989;**43**:227-232

[36] Bai R, Wan L, Li H, Zhang Z, Ma Z. Identify the injury implements by SEM/EDX and ICP-AES. Forensic Science International. 2007;**166**:8-13. DOI: 10.1016/j.forsciint.2006.03.008

[37] Tanaka N, Aga F, Takakura A, Jamal M, Ito A, Kumihashi M, et al. An autopsy case of retained an oil-based contrast medium. Forensic Pathology. 2017;**23**:29-32

[38] Tanaka N, Aga F, Takakura A, Jamal M, Tsutsui K, Kamo K, et al. Barium retention. Forensic Pathology. 2018;**24**:57-60

[39] Saukko P, Knight B. Knight's Forensic Pathology. 3rd ed. London: Hodder Arnold; 2004

[40] Tanaka N, Kinoshita H, Takakura A, Wakabayashi A, Sudo H, Okano K, et al. Application of energy dispersive X-ray fluorescence spectrometry (EDX) for the identification of a foreign body. Review of Albanian Legal Medicine. 2016;**12**:67-71

[41] Winstanley R, Patel I, Fischer E. The determination of toxic metals in simulated stomach contents by energy dispersive X-ray fluorescence analysis and a fatal case of mercury poisoning. Forensic Science International. 1987;**35**:181-187. DOI: 10.1016/0379-0738(87)90054-5

[42] Ozo Y, Yoshizawa M, Murata A, Shimazaki S, Kajiwara M, Takagi T, et al. Simple quantitation of arsenic by energy dispersive fluorescence X-ray spectrometer using Reinsch's test. Chūdoku Kenkyū. 2004;**17**:359-364

[43] Tanaka N, Takakura A, Kumihashi M, Jamal M, Ito A, Kimura S, et al. Applicability of energy dispersive X-ray fluorescence spectrometry (EDX) for arsenic identification in stomach contents. Current Study Environmental Medicine Science. 2017;**10**:10-13

[44] Tanaka N, Kinoshita H, Takakura A, Jamal M, Kumihashi M, Uchiyama Y, et al. Combination of energy-dispersive X-ray fluorescence spectrometry (EDX) and head-space gas chromatography

mass spectrometry (HS-GC/MS) is a useful screening tool for stomach contents. Romanian Journal of Legal Medicine. 2015;**23**:43-44. DOI: 10.4323/rjlm.2015.43

[45] Kinoshita H, Tanaka N, Jamal M, Kumihashi M, Okuzono R, Tsutsui K, et al. Application of energy dispersive X-ray fluorescence spectrometry (EDX) in a case of methomyl ingestion. Forensic Science International. 2013;**227**:103-105. DOI: 10.1016/j.forsciint.2012.08.026

[46] Takahashi M, Kinoshita H, Nishiguchi M, Kasuda S, Ouchi H, Minami T, et al. Application of energy dispersive X-ray fluorescent spectrometry (EDXRF) in drug related cases. Legal Medicine. 2009;**11**(Supplement 1):S411-S412. DOI: 10.1016/j.legalmed.2009.01.077

[47] Takahashi M, Kinoshita H, Kuse A, Morichika M, Nishiguchi M, Ouchi H, et al. Application of energy dispersive X-ray fluorescence spectrometry (EDX) in medico-legal autopsy case. In: Vieira DN, Busuttil A, Cusack D, Beth P, editors. Acta Medicinae Legalis et Socialis. Coimbra: Coimbra University Press; 2010. pp. 325-328

[48] Kinoshita H, Tanaka N, Kumihashi M, Jamal M, Takakura A, Umemoto T, et al. Titanium in stomach contents—Does it provide useful information for forensic diagnosis? Romanian Journal of Legal Medicine. 2014;**22**:117-118. DOI: 10.4323/rjlm.2014.117

[49] Sugibayashi K, editor. Zukai Seizaigaku. Nanzando: Tokyo; 2013

[50] Tanaka N, Takakura A, Kumihashi M, Jamal M, Ito A, Kimura S, et al. Application of energy-dispersive X-ray fluorescence spectrometry (EDX) in forensics—Titanium, silicon and

magnesium in the stomach contents as good indicators for ingestion of pharmaceutical tablets. Romanian Journal of Legal Medicine. 2017;**25**:89-91. DOI: 10.4323/rjlm.2017.89

[51] Tanaka N, Kinoshita H, Takakura A, Ohbayashi Y, Jamal M, Ameno K. Forensic odontological application for dental restorations in case of skeletal remains using energy-dispersive X-ray fluorescence spectrometry. Albanian Journal of Medical and Health Sciences. 2018;**49**:1-4

[52] Yamashita H, Tanaka N, Ikemastsu K, Kinoshita H. Application of elemental analysis by energy-dispersive X-ray fluorescence spectrometry (EDX) to dental restorations: Improved sampling using a steel bur and cotton swab. New Bulletin of Medical Science. 2020;**4**(2):3-6

Chapter 4

Forensic Dentistry

Nihal Yetimoğlu

Abstract

In forensic science, forensic dentistry has become a crucial component that helps identify deceased people who cannot be identified visually or through other means. Dental records are inspected and assessed before presentation in the interest of justice and the law. Identification is difficult in medicolegal cases where people's responses are erroneous or misleading, making it difficult to draw the correct conclusions. Digital forensics has replaced traditional forensic investigations in acquiring, analyzing, and reporting forensic evidence. A definition of digital forensics might be "the use of computer science and investigative techniques for a legal purpose involving the analysis of digital evidence." Traditional written dental records are subject to subjectivity in their creation and analysis, which leaves them open to mistakes and omissions when identifying unidentified bodies. The authors recommend digitizing and standardizing dental records to improve the dependability of these analog techniques. A machine's ability to mimic human intelligence and behavior to carry out particular tasks is known as artificial intelligence (AI). AI has advanced rapidly in recent years and could be helpful for efficient forensic dental identification.

Keywords: forensic dentistry, age determination, sex determination, intraoral scanners, artificial intelligence

1. Introduction

Because of its historical significance, the study of forensic dentistry must continue to advance. A dental forensic investigation may involve identifying a single person or, in certain situations, several people, such as in mass disasters. In the latter case, forensic pathologists, forensic odontologists, and forensic anthropologists would work together to perform biological profiling and population stratification [1].

Multiple-fatality stratification is the process of grouping people according to their age, with sex and ethnic background playing a minor role. The likelihood of positively identifying a missing person from their dental records is increased when this procedure is used on a collection of unidentified human remains [1]. In the absence of identification, the forensic dentist may ascertain chronological age by evaluating the developmental age of a person's dentition through diagnostic imaging. The use of digital technologies, particularly technological advances, has significantly enhanced dental and medical procedures, especially in the visualization of treatment targets and diagnoses. These advancements could further improve clinical practices in forensic dentistry and forensic medicine.

Visual comparisons between antemortem dental records and postmortem findings have been the primary technique used in forensic dentistry to identify individuals. The combination of decayed, missing, and filled teeth in forensic settings makes the dentition unique [2]. Because teeth are so resilient—they can withstand high temperatures and decomposition—postmortem dental examinations are essential for identifying a person, even under challenging circumstances. Although each person has roughly the same number of teeth, each person's teeth differ in size, shape, form, and color [3].

Multiple-fatality stratification classifies people according to age and, to a lesser degree, sex and ethnic background. Applying this procedure to a collection of unidentified human remains raises the likelihood that a missing person's dental records will be positively identified. If identification is not feasible, the forensic dentist may be able to ascertain chronological age and sex by utilizing diagnostic imaging to evaluate the developmental age of a person's dentition.

Legal authorities can identify victims and suspects with the help of easily readable dental records, including radiographs, cast models, digital dental impressions, clinical photos, patient information, and pathological reports, among many others [1]. In addition to having a solid understanding of general dentistry, which includes all dental specialties, the forensic odontologist should also be familiar with the fundamentals of autopsy procedures and the function of forensic pathologists. When comparing the antemortem and postmortem reports, it is essential to observe any similarities and differences.

2. Age estimation

Determining the victim's or the remains' sex and estimating their age at death are crucial guidelines that aid in the identification process. The significance of age estimation in medicolegal and anthropological contexts encompasses criminal cases, judicial punishments, marriage, employment, kidnapping, rape, and many other situations.

Age estimation is aided by volumetric analysis of dental features in radiographs, such as pulpal size reduction, which results in the formation of secondary dentin since secondary dentin deposition is proportionate to an individual's age.

Age estimation can be divided into three stages:

2.1 Neonatal, postnatal, and antenatal

The prenatal jawbones, the appearance of tooth germs, the early mineralization of primary teeth during intrauterine life, and the degree of crown completion determine the prenatal, neonatal, and postnatal phases.

2.2 Adolescents and children

The earliest discernible sign of tooth mineralization, the degree of crown completion, the eruption time of a tooth in the oral cavity, the degree of root completion of erupted and/or unerupted teeth, the degree of root resorption of deciduous teeth, the presence of open apices in teeth, and the appearance of tooth germs are the basis for this phase.

2.3 Adult

This includes evaluating the pulp volume of teeth and the development of third molars.

Also, according to Harvey [1], the following elements could help determine dental age:

- The way tooth germs look

- The first observable sign of mineralization

- The extent of the unerupted tooth's completion

- Rate of enamel formation and neonatal line formation

- Clinical eruption

- Degree of root completion of teeth that have erupted

- Deciduous tooth resorption degree

- Attrition of the crown

- Physiologic secondary dentin formation

- Cementum formation

- Openness of the root dentine

- Gingival recession

- Root surface resorption

- Discoloration and staining of teeth

- Changes in the chemical composition of the teeth

- Influence of disease or malnutrition on tooth eruption

- Influence of sex on tooth eruption.

Age can be determined by physical, chemical, radiographic, histological, clinical, or visual examination, depending on the method of inquiry.

3. Sexual determination

Forensic specialists find it extremely difficult to determine sex from skeletal remains, mainly when only pieces of the body are found. Forensic dentists can help other specialists identify the sex of the remains by analyzing skulls and teeth [1, 4].

Male and female sexes differ in a number of tooth characteristics, including morphology, crown size, and root lengths. The most commonly measured dental factors for determining sex are the dimensions of permanent teeth, such as the mesiodistal size. Because they exhibit the most pronounced sexual dimorphism in their dimensions, canines are considered a "key tooth" in sex determination and have been used consistently for forensic purposes among various tooth types [5]. Males have larger tooth crowns than females in modern human populations, though this difference varies by population.

Additionally, there are variations in the patterns of the skull and mandible. One of the most potent craniofacial bones for gender identification, according to the literature, is the mandible [4, 6]. Its safe components for sex determination are found in its morphological variation and relative indestructibility. Some mandibular measurements exhibit sexual dimorphism, according to a prior systematic review that assessed a number of mandibular parameters investigated for sexual dimorphism. Adult cranial analysis methods for determining sex are already well-established and show excellent accuracy. It has been demonstrated that an individual's sex has a significant impact on their cranial, facial, nasal, and maxillary widths.

4. Digital dental records

Digital dental records, also known as dental charts, are official documents that include all of the patient's medical history, current condition, clinical examination, diagnosis, treatment, and prognosis [7]. Preserved digital evidence is essential for in-person identification, particularly when it comes to disaster victim identification, where there are many victims, the bodies are severely disfigured or mutilated, and the only source of victim identification is dental tissues. In order to protect patients' best interests and ensure the continuity and safety of their dental care, dentists are required by law and professional standards to keep accurate dental records [8]. Digital records should be electronically stored for a minimum of 7 to 10 years. It is created using digital images of the patient's mouth and dental data. Rapid comparison of the AM and PM records of deceased victims in the event of terrorism, earthquakes, mass disasters, etc., are made possible by computerized software. Additionally, digital radiographs and photos of the deceased can be superimposed and compared using software. These online dental records will serve as a valuable source of proof for body identification in the ensuing decades.

5. Digital radiography for forensics

In forensic examinations, digital radiographs are crucial because they offer unbiased proof of the anatomical conditions and dental procedures performed up to that point. They are advantageous because they are quick, easy, and nondestructive ways to obtain information. They are also more cost-effective than DNA technology. Digital radiography is very beneficial because it makes it possible to compare antemortem and postmortem radiographs side by side with better image quality, which speeds up the identification process. Additionally, images can be instantly displayed on the computer screen and enhanced for optimal viewing (**Figures 1–3**).

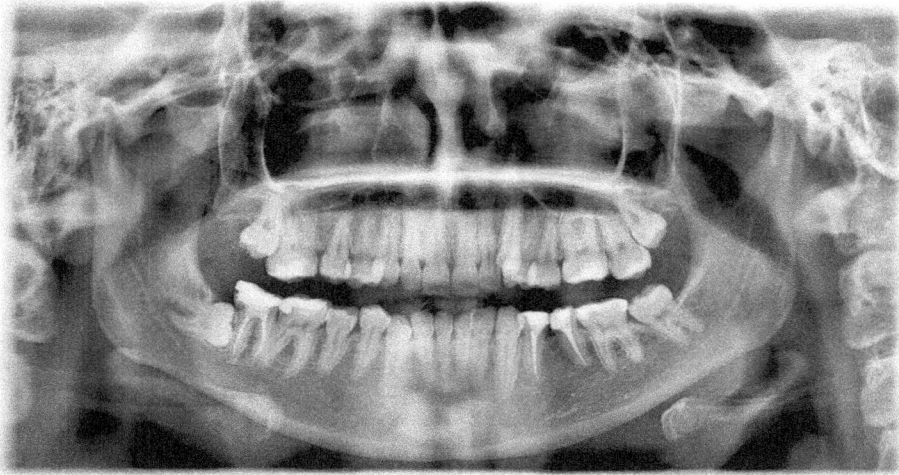

Figure 1.
Digital panoramic radiograph.

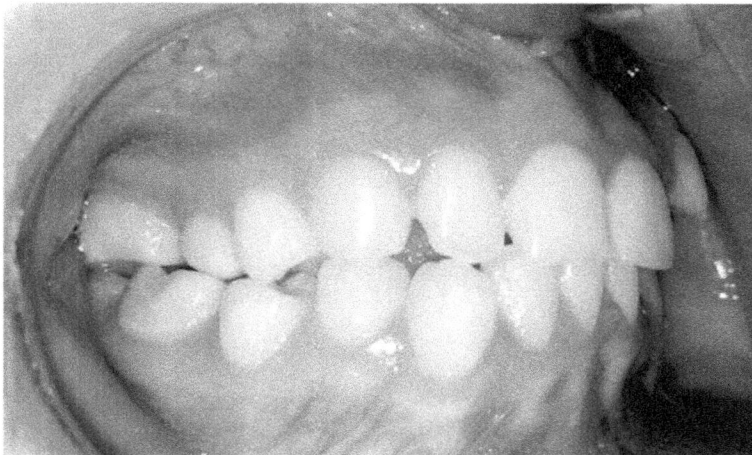

Figure 2.
Recording obtained using an intraoral scanner.

Finding the concordant points for positive or potential identification involves comparing the AM and PM radiographs of the maxillofacial and dental structures. Numerous dental findings—such as the presence or absence of teeth, development of a third molar, extra teeth, a tooth's crown and root structure, pulpal anatomy, decayed and restored teeth, endodontic treatment, and prosthetic treatment, to mention a few—are used to evaluate these data. An identification occurs when there are enough distinguishing characteristics between the AM and PM data that are the same with comprehensible differences. Since the most recent films will most closely resemble the postmortem condition of the teeth and jaws, they are analyzed first. A comparison is made with Ref. [9].

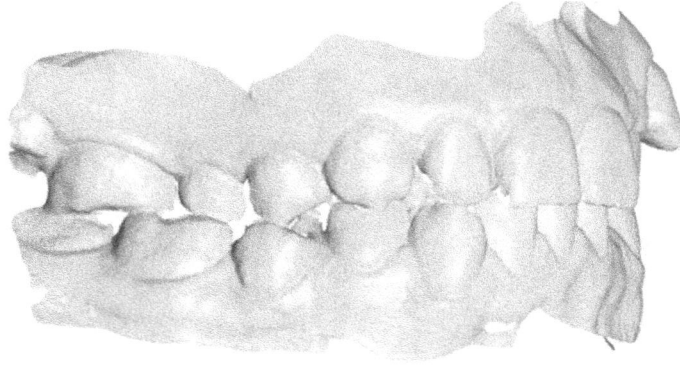

Figure 3.
Recording obtained using an intraoral scanner.

- Number and arrangement of teeth (missing teeth, rotated teeth, spacing, extra teeth, impacted teeth

- Caries and periodontal bone loss

- Coronal restorations

- Hidden restorations (posts, implants, root canal fillings)

- Bony pathology

- Dental anatomy

- Trabecular bone pattern

- Anatomic bony landmarks

- Maxillary sinus and nasal aperture

- Frontal sinus

Recently, CBCT has allowed for precise examination of the spatial relationships of dental structures, such as teeth, roots, and supporting structures, on AM and PM images and accurate alignment between AM and PM radiographs without additional exposures. Furthermore, it helps reconstructive technology create a biological profile of a deceased or missing individual whose identity is unknown.

6. Digital photography in bite marks

In forensic cases, photography is the most effective way to gather and preserve evidence, particularly regarding bite mark analysis and human abuse cases. Bite marks are wounds or indentations on skin or objects brought on by teeth, either by themselves or in conjunction with another oral anatomy. Bite marks typically include superficial abrasion, subsurface hemorrhage, or skin bruising due to the bite [10]. The forensic department finds it difficult to analyze and compare bite marks because of the numerous combinations caused by tissue elasticity, jaw movements, impression distortion, or flawed photography, among other factors. Bite marks come in seven different varieties [1]:

- Hemorrhage (a small bleeding spot)

- Abrasion (undamaging mark on skin)

- Contusion (ruptured blood vessels, bruise)

- Laceration (near puncture of skin)

- Incision (neatly punctured or torn skin)

- Avulsion (removal of skin)

- Artifact (a bitten-off piece of body)

It is essential to take precise pictures of the injuries because these serve as a permanent record of the victim's injuries, and they are necessary for comparing the suspect's dentition to the bite mark injury.

Digital cameras take pictures, which are then digitalized by the camera's sensor and transformed into computerized image files. Images can be saved to the computer, where they can be edited, sent by email, or printed as needed. Bitmapped images, such as JPEG, PNG, TIFF, GIF, and BMP, and vector-based images created with "pain in drawing" or "illustration" programs primarily concentrating on image manipulation or enhancement are the two categories of digital images.

To improve the appearance of damage in situations where the skin is disrupted, nonvisible photography—which uses infrared and ultraviolet light—was introduced. It captures the specifics of bite mark injuries on skin that appear fully healed when exposed to visible light. Biting causes significant damage to the skin's surface and the subepithelial surface, which leads to subdermal hemorrhage.

7. Intraoral three-dimensional optical scanners

Using intraoral scanners to scan the dental arch, directly and indirectly, has significantly increased bite mark impression accuracy. A probe with a sapphire or hard steel tip is used by 3D contact (point-to-point or linear) scanners to analyze an object's surface [11]. The main limitation is the longer time to conduct point-to-point scanning; it requires physical contact with the object, and it becomes challenging to scan concave surfaces. This could be avoided by using laser or optical scanners, which use laser light to scan an object's surface, such as the occlusal details of the teeth in the dental arch. A 3D surface model is produced by triangulating the multiple point clouds that are made at various locations by the scanning software after the sensor's images have been further processed. The available bite mark evidence can be compared to these 3D images. Anterior tooth

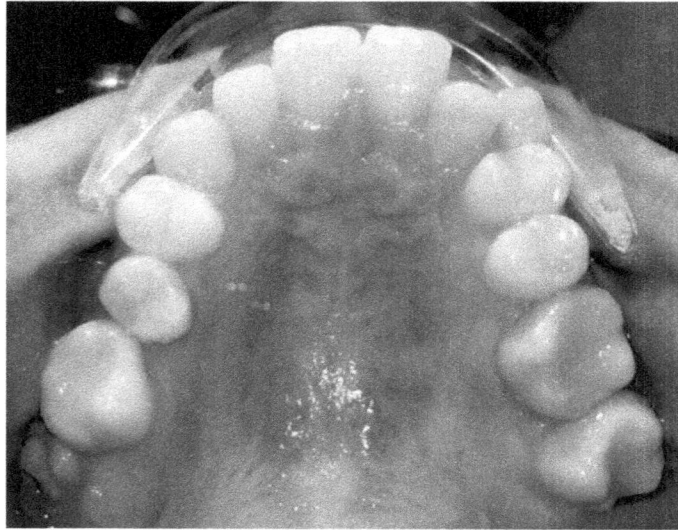

Figure 4.
Recording obtained using an intraoral scanner.

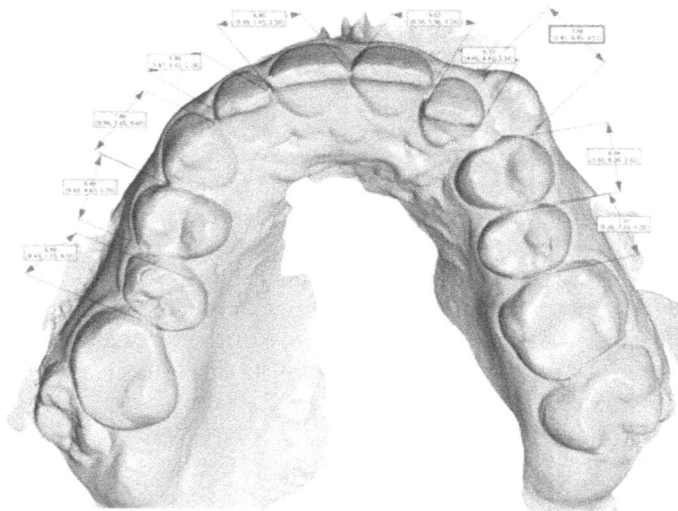

Figure 5.
Recording obtained using an intraoral scanner.

width, thickness, spacing, intercanine distance, rotational and labiolingual tooth positions, indications of tooth misalignment in the arch, and biting edge curves should all be assessed (**Figures 4** and **5**).

8. Cheiloscopy

The red mucosa of the lips, also known as Klein's zone, is covered in several lines, furrows, and lip wrinkles that differ in quantity, thickness, length, ramification, and location [12]. These combinations of variations provide a distinct lip pattern for every individual. The lips create a specific mark, the lip print when they contact a surface. At the crime scene, it can be found on clothing, windows, doors, cigarettes, glasses, and cups. These lip prints were created during the sixth month of intrauterine life and are genetic. Even after death, it remains distinct, unalterable, and permanent. There are various lip-print classifications [13].

Suzuki and Tsuchihashi's classification of lip prints:

Type I: Vertical, clear-cut grooves that span the whole lip.

Type I^1: Not covering the entire lip but like Type I.

Type II: Grooves with branches.

Type III: Intersected grooves.

Type IV: Reticular grooves.

Type V: grooves that cannot be morphologically differentiated.

Martin Santos classification:

This author divides the lip grooves into two groups:

1. Simple: several elements form an element; this element can be a straight line (R-1), a curve (C-2), an angular form (A-3), or a sinusoidal (S-4)

2. compound, when several elements form them; in this case, they can be bifurcated (B-5), trifurcated (T-6), or anomalous (An-7).

Renaud classification:

This is the most comprehensive classification. The left and right lips are examined in pairs, and each groove is assigned a number based on its shape (**Table 1**). After that, a formula is developed that uses capital letters to describe the left (L) and right (R) sides of the upper lip and small letters to categorize each groove. For the lower lip, the opposite is true, with small letters being used to distinguish between the left and right sides and capital letters to categorize the grooves.

Afchar-Bayat classification:

As shown in **Table 2**, this 1979 classification is based on a six-type groove organization.

Classification	Groove type
A	Complete vertical
B	Incomplete vertical
C	Complete bifurcated
D	Incomplete bifurcated
E	Completely branched
F	Incomplete branched
G	Reticular pattern
H	X or coma form
I	Horizontal
J	Other forms (ellipse, triangle)

Table 1.
Renaud lip prints classification.

Classification	Groove type
A1	Vertical and straight grooves covering the whole lip
A2	Like the former, but not covering the whole lip
B1	Straight branched grooves
B2	Angulated branched groove
C	Converging grooves
D	Reticular pattern grooves
E	Other grooves

Table 2.
Jose´ Maria Dominguez classification.

This categorization is based on the Suzuki and Tsuchihashi classification. The author and his colleagues noticed a slight variation in the grooves classified as Type II by Suzuki and Tsuchihashi. They saw that branched grooves frequently divided downward in the lower lip and upward in the upper lip, as reported by Suzuki and Tsuchihashi. However, they also realized that some grooves, the so-called II0 type, branched the opposite way.

9. Palatoscopy

The oral mucosa's surface is smooth and flat, devoid of crests or grooves [12]. This is done to maximize oral function performance. However, some exceptions do exist: the papillae that cover the back of the tongue and the anterior region of the palatal mucosa, which has a thick network of rugae that are securely affixed to the underlying bone.

The ridges on the palate's anterior surface that extend bilaterally from the mid-palatine raphae behind the incisive papilla are known as palatal rugae. Their functions include aiding chewing, preventing food loss from the mouth, and facilitating food movement through the oral cavity.

The hard connective tissue that covers the bone forms palatal rugae during the third month of pregnancy. Once formed, they only change in length due to normal growth, staying in the same place for the duration of a person's life. These rugae are well protected by lips, cheeks, alveolus, teeth, and tongue during high-impact trauma, assaults, mass disasters, and fire accidents. Using the software, the rugae are compared to the digital impression, cone-beam computed tomography (CBCT), dental cast, and earlier photos from the dental records.

Palatal rugae are currently classified into several different categories. Nonetheless, several authors claim that Lysell created the first classification scheme for palatal rugae pairs in 1955 [14]. Analysis of palatal rugae can be done in several ways. Intraoral inspection is the most popular, simplest, and least expensive method. It may cause problems if a subsequent comparative test is necessary.

The three-dimensional, digitalized palate acquired from intraoral scanners enables the development of an automatic pattern recognition technique using artificial intelligence and highly accurate geometrical measurements. When the identification was done by visual classification of palatal rugae, the former method could be eliminated by superimposing palatal scans and computing surface deviation.

10. Artificial intelligence in forensic dentistry

The ability of a machine to mimic human intelligence and behavior to carry out particular tasks is known as artificial intelligence (AI) [15, 16]. AI has developed quickly in recent years and has had a significant impact on people's lifestyles. Numerous artificial intelligence (AI) technologies, including virtual assistants, image recognition, and online search engines, have helped people's daily lives and enhanced their quality of life. AI development and application have also surfaced in the medical field. AI technology has the possibility of improving patient care through better diagnostic aids and reduced errors in daily practice.

Given the extensive use of artificial intelligence in both medicine and law, where it is currently frequently employed to locate pertinent records and evidence in court cases, it makes sense to anticipate that forensic medicine and forensic dentistry will also use this. Technology. Deep neural networks, artificial neural networks, machine learning, and computer technology are examples of artificial intelligence-based technologies utilized in forensic dentistry. Artificial intelligence can advance forensic dentistry in numerous ways, such as dental identification. By analyzing dental images, including radiographs, artificial intelligence can assist forensic dentists in matching and identifying individuals based on their jaws and teeth [17].

- Estimating age and sex: Forensic dentists can use artificial intelligence to analyze dental images and determine a person's age and sex.

- Facial reconstruction: Artificial intelligence can produce 3D models of teeth and jaws and reconstruct the faces of unidentified remains.

- Bite mark analysis: Artificial intelligence can analyze and match bite marks that may be used as evidence in criminal cases.

- Dental databases: Artificial intelligence can be used to search and match dental data in databases to ascertain a person's identity.

- Chatbots: Artificial intelligence-driven chatbots can help people learn about forensic dentistry and get answers to their questions.

- Task automation: By automating specific processes, like dental image analysis, artificial intelligence can decrease the need for manual labor and improve identification speed and accuracy.

Artificial intelligence can estimate a person's age by analyzing images of their face, teeth, or bones, among other features. It can also evaluate dental images, including x-rays, and determine an individual's age by analyzing the growth and wear of their teeth. AI can create predictive models that use various data, including measurements, photos, and demographic data, to determine an individual's age, sex, and dental identification.

11. Conclusions

In conclusion, we can presume that the AI feature will change the way forensic dentistry is practiced in all areas, including sex determination and age estimation. As a useful tool for future research and even routine forensic analyses, experts are now being guided into the era of artificial intelligence. Advanced AI implementation still necessitates interdisciplinary collaboration, but with comprehension.

Acknowledgements

The author would like to thank Prof. Dr. M. Haluk İşeri for all the support given.

Conflict of interest

The author declares no conflict of interest.

Author details

Nihal Yetimoğlu
Faculty of Dentistry, Maxillofacial Radiology, Istanbul Yeniyuzyil University, Istanbul, Turkey

*Address all correspondence to: nihal.yetimoglu@yeniyuzyil.edu.tr

IntechOpen

References

[1] Jayakrishnan JM, Reddy J, Vinod Kumar RB. Role of forensic odontology and anthropology in the identification of human remains. Journal of Oral and Maxillofacial Pathology. 2021;**25**(3):543-547. DOI: 10.4103/jomfp.jomfp_81_21. Epub 2022 Jan 11

[2] Matsuda S, Yoshida H, Ebata K, Shimada I, Yoshimura H. Forensic odontology with digital technologies: A systematic review. Journal of Forensic and Legal Medicine. 2020;**74**:102004. DOI: 10.1016/j.jflm.2020.102004. Epub 2020 Jul 1

[3] Prakash P, Singh MK, Bhandari SK. Forensic odontology: The prosthetic ID. Journal of Forensic Dental Sciences. 2019;**11**(3):113-117. DOI: 10.4103/jfo. jfds_91_19. Epub 2020 Jun 3

[4] de Araujo CM, de Jesus Freitas PF, Ferraz AX, Quadras ICC, Zeigelboim BS, Priolo Filho S, et al. Sex determination through the maxillary dental arch and skeletal base measurements using machine learning. Head & Face Medicine. 2024;**20**(1):44. DOI: 10.1186/s13005-024-00446-w

[5] Tajik M, Movahhedian N. Canine sexual dimorphism in crown and root dimensions: A cone-beam computed tomographic study. The Journal of Forensic Odonto-Stomatology. 2024;**42**(1):12-21. DOI: 10.5281/zenodo.11061431

[6] Küchler EC, Kirschneck C, Marañón-Vásquez GA, Schroder ÂGD, Baratto-Filho F, Romano FL, et al. Mandibular and dental measurements for sex determination using machine learning. Scientific Reports. 2024;**14**(1):9587. DOI: 10.1038/s41598-024-59556-9

[7] Nagi R, Aravinda K, Rakesh N, Jain S, Kaur N, Mann AK. Digitization in forensic odontology: A paradigm shift in forensic investigations. Journal of Forensic Dental Sciences. 2019;**11**(1):5-10. DOI: 10.4103/jfo. jfds_55_19

[8] Al-Azri AR, Harford J, James H. Awareness of forensic odontology among dentists in Australia: Are they keeping forensically valuable dental records? Australian Dental Journal. 2016;**61**(1):102-108. DOI: 10.1111/adj.12316. Epub 2016 Feb 10

[9] Manigandan T, Sumathy C, Elumalai M, Sathasivasubramanian S, Kannan A. Forensic radiology in dentistry. Journal of Pharmacy & Bioallied Sciences. 2015;**7**(Suppl. 1):S260-S264. DOI: 10.4103/0975-7406.155944

[10] Verma AK, Kumar S, Rathore S, Pandey A. Role of a dental expert in forensic odontology. National Journal of Maxillofacial Surgery. 2014;**5**(1):2-5. DOI: 10.4103/0975-5950.140147

[11] Simon B, Lipták L, Lipták K, Tárnoki ÁD, Tárnoki DL, Melicher D, et al. Application of intraoral scanner to identify monozygotic twins. BMC Oral Health. 2020;**20**(1):268. DOI: 10.1186/s12903-020-01261-w

[12] Chaves T, Azevedo Á, Caldas IM. Cheiloscopy in sex estimation: A systematic review. Forensic Science, Medicine, and Pathology. 2024;**20**(1):280-292. DOI: 10.1007/s12024-023-00648-9. Epub 2023 May 27

[13] Caldas IM, Magalhães T, Afonso A. Establishing identity using cheiloscopy and palatoscopy. Forensic Science International. 2007;**165**(1):1-9.

DOI: 10.1016/j.forsciint.2006.04.010.
Epub 2006 May 24

[14] Jain A, Chowdhary R. Palatal
rugae and their role in forensic
odontology. Journal of Investigative and
Clinical Dentistry. 2014;**5**(3):171-178.
DOI: 10.1111/j.2041-1626.2013.00150.x.
Epub 2013 Feb 1

[15] Vodanović M, Subašić M,
Milošević DP, Galić I, Brkić H. Artificial
intelligence in forensic medicine
and forensic dentistry. The Journal
of Forensic Odonto-Stomatology.
2023;**41**(2):30-41

[16] Putra RH, Doi C, Yoda N, Astuti ER,
Sasaki K. Current applications and
development of artificial intelligence
for digital dental radiography.
Dento Maxillo Facial Radiology.
2022;**51**(1):20210197. DOI: 10.1259/
dmfr.20210197. Epub 2021 Jul 8

[17] Bui R, Iozzino R, Richert R, Roy P,
Boussel L, Tafrount C, et al. Artificial
intelligence as a decision-making tool
in forensic dentistry: A pilot study
with I3M. International Journal of
Environmental Research and Public
Health. 2023;**20**(5):4620. DOI: 10.3390/
ijerph20054620

Chapter 5

Forensic Anthropology in Aircraft Disasters: The Cuban Experience

Dodany Machado Mendoza

Abstract

This chapter addresses the importance of forensic anthropological work in identifying victims in situations of aircraft disasters, catastrophic events where trauma is severe and the bodies are often burned to death, with the consequent destruction of the same. Elements are provided on the Cuban experience in these situations, methodologies and protocols used. It also describes how a particular closed disaster was handled, the 883 Aerocaribbean aircraft disaster, where practically all the bodies were charred and reduced to only fragments. The importance of teamwork and the work at the scene of the accident facilitated the identification of all the deceased in that plane.

Keywords: catastrophe, aircraft, identification, forensic work, anthropologist

1. Introduction

Forensic Anthropology is nothing more than the application of anthropological knowledge for justice and society. Forensic anthropologist in their daily work faces various issues, and the most common is the identification of human remains, skeletonized, or in decomposition's stage, when simple identification methods are not viable (facial recognition and fingerprints analysis, among others). The objective of identification is to arrive at the identity of the corpse(s) or human remains [1].

Forensic anthropologists work at the request of a competent authority, as required by legal action. Also, the study of injuries, especially bone, that could have caused death or be related to the dynamics of a criminal act. Likewise, the study of the products of conception (fetuses) for the determination of gestational age and bone lesions that may be related to illegal abortions or infanticides. However, the greatest work is linked to the investigation of cadaveric remains, for example, in aircraft disasters with a lot of cadavers.

It is necessary to point out that in this science, there will always be a counterpart that makes the researcher more demanding. The deceased have acquaintances, relatives, friends, people who interacted with them, and records of any kind, among other aspects, that help to corroborate their identification.

2. Forensic anthropology in disasters

The United Nations Office for Disaster Risk Reduction (UNISDR) defines a disaster (or catastrophe) as "a serious disruption in the functioning of a community or society that causes a large number of deaths, as well as losses and impacts material, economic and environmental, that exceed the capacity of the affected community or society to face the situation through the use of their own resources" [2].

From the forensic point of view, several definitions arise. Vallejo and Alonso define a catastrophe as "an event characterized by being an unexpected, unusual event, of rapid onset, of a collective nature, which produces material and human destruction and for whose resolution the intervention of extraordinary aid means is necessary, both by their number and by their nature" [3].

The Royal College of Pathologists defines it as "an episode in which the number of deaths exceeds that which can be dealt with by the use of normal resources, particularly as regards the mortuary" [4]. In Cuba, it is managed as an event, whether natural or anthropic, that exceeds the ability to respond to the community.

The Emergency Events Database (EM-DAT) classifies catastrophes into two broad categories, according to their origin: natural and technological. These are in turn divided into subgroups, types and subtypes. For example, a natural catastrophe can be of geophysical origin (earthquakes), meteorological (hurricanes, tornadoes), hydrological (floods), climatological (droughts), biological (epidemics) or extraterrestrial (meteorite impact). On the other hand, technological catastrophes can be from an industrial, transport or other type of accident linked to anthropic events [5].

Although these subdivisions exist, the two major categories can be related and one can trigger the other, as occurs with seismic events that produce major technological impacts (e.g., the earthquake in Japan in 2011 and its subsequent tsunami, which caused damage to the Fukushima nuclear power plant, with the release of radioactive material).

The WHO incorporates a chronological criterion and distinguishes between emergencies that occur suddenly, with a greater forensic interest (such as earthquakes, meteorological events and air disasters) and those that develop slowly (droughts) [6]. Other situations can be more complex, such as war conflicts, civil conflicts and mass displacement of people in shipwrecks, for example. In these cases, working conditions are more difficult due to both the political situation and security issues [7].

La Guía de Interpol de Identificación de Víctimas de Catástrofes (IVC), refleja la importancia de distinguir también las catástrofes en abiertas o cerradas, ya que esto influye en la forma de trabajo y el tipo de respuesta en término de identificación de las víctimas [8]. None disaster is like another, and the effectiveness of the work will often depend on the experience of the specialists, as well as the working and management conditions.

The identification of victims of major catastrophes is carried out based on the evaluation of multiple factors. The degree of deterioration of the corpses, the time they have been exposed to the elements and the changes they experience, aspects that affect the possibility of applying specific identification methods. For this purpose, work protocols in disasters are used as well as the guides of Interpol and the International Committee of the Red Cross [9].

Identification methods used in disasters must be scientifically valid, reliable and applicable within a reasonable period of time, for existing conditions on the ground. The primary and most reliable means of identification are comparative dental analysis, fingerprinting, and DNA profiling. Secondary media include personal description and medical data, as well as clues and clothing associated with the body. These means serve to reinforce the identification established in another way and, generally, by themselves, are not enough to certify it.

All possible methods should be used. Identification based only on photographs is not absolute and should be avoided at all costs. Visual identification by a witness can be useful, but it is not sufficient for the identification of victims of major disasters, since they have often suffered so much trauma that visual comparison is impossible and, moreover, family members are often unable to cope with the psychological pressure of seeing deceased victims. All postmortem data obtained from the corpses are compared with reference to the information available about the absence.

In disasters, depending on the magnitude, the same can be found in intact corpses, as fragmented, and on many occasions, if there were fires or explosions, burned or charred, so the identification methods are somewhat affected. Fingerprints cannot be collected; the bursting of the skull means that teeth are not possessed, dismemberment, etc. The application of Forensic Anthropology methods in cases of deaths in disaster situations is extremely important, mainly in those cases in which identification through simple inspection is impossible.

3. Aircraft disasters: The place of catastrophe

The place of the accident can vary greatly, from those that occur at sea, to the impact on a mountain or the explosion in mid-flight. Depending on it will be the degree of complexity.

In a disaster at sea, despite the fact that most of the bodies are generally lost, what it has in favor is that there is no prolonged fire, since the water puts it out. The mountain brings with it the difficult process of accessing, investigating the place, and transferring the bodies and the work personnel, while the explosion in the air includes scattering of the bodies and parts of the aircraft, especially at high altitudes, as occurred with the space shuttle "Columbia."

To work in the place of disaster does not always come on the same day as the catastrophe, sometimes wait for days because the place is in fire, or the air is contaminated, or simply the access is difficult. The forensic anthropologist must go to the scene of the accident, especially when it occurs in a place with a hot and humid climate with multiple victims, since this delays the process of arrival at the place, fixation, measurement, survey, packaging and transfer, of the bodies, these can decompose or be altered, and there are elements of identity that can be detected at the scene of the accident that is not appreciated later in the morgue. Therefore, it is important to photographically fix everything that identifies it and locate it topographically, with respect to the position on the site and that of the corpse in its context.

In lifting, clothing and other objects are considered to belong to the individual if they have anatomical continuity with the individual. Loose body parts are considered to belong to another subject if they are not connected to the body by at least a fragment of tissue.

This action has to be carried out with the appropriate light and the necessary means, and it does not end until all the parts of the corpse are located, which is not always possible due to the taphonomic events that may have occurred: dispersal by scavengers, corpse in aquatic environment (sea streams), being located on an inclined plane (hill and mountain), dispersal by the rescue of survivors.

After being fixed photographically, with video or sketches of the place of discovery, and after collecting all the available parts of the corpses, it is packed correctly and the packaging is labeled for transfer and study in the forensic medical entity or the place assigned for this work.

4. Identification of bodies or fragments

After the bodies or parts have been rescued, the classification work corresponds. The classification is nothing more than the determination of the identifying tetralogy of each fragment or part that was collected, which is nothing more than the determination of the sex, the ancestral pattern, the height and the age that the subject(s) must have had at death; also known as "Big Four." The quality with which it is made and the accuracy will later determine the speed with which the identifications are achieved.

Sex determination is based on the sexual dimorphism present in the human species. If the corpses or fragments did not include the external genitals, we used other methods. In a general sense, male are more robust and their diameters and circumferences are larger. On the other hand, as a product of evolution, the female pelvis has undergone important changes for adaptation to pregnancy, from the bipedal posture being the most dimorphic region for sexual differentiation.

In terms of ancestral pattern, it is currently divided into three main groups: Whites (European ancestors), Blacks (Sub-Saharan African and Australoid ancestors), Mongoloid (East Asian and Amerindian ancestors) and a mixture of these groups. If the skin, hair or face not exist, the main differences are located in the skull and face, with very specific characteristics of each ancestral pattern, although as cosmopolitan biological beings and with interactions between groups, these patterns are not so strict. What arises is the skull has predominant characteristics of a determined ancestral pattern.

The height from human remains is calculated taking into account regression equations obtained for the different populations from studies carried out in them, which are mainly based on the lengths of the long bones or their fragments. It is recommended that equations calculated from each population be used in order to have more accuracy when estimating.

To calculate the age, it is first verified whether the remains correspond to a subadult or an adult. If it is a subadult, the method is based on the analysis of the stage of growth and development in which it is found (X-rays are very useful). As life progresses until approximately 28 years of age, growth changes occur in the skeleton; first, ossification points appear, and then the epiphyses begin to fuse with the diaphyses. The order in which each process occurs is reported in the dissimilar investigations carried out on the subject. Likewise, dental evolution has been studied in the same way.

When the subject is already "osteologically" an adult, then the age is calculated by the deterioration that the person suffers over the course of life. There are regions of the body that present gradual changes that are well studied and are closely related to the environmental effects of climate, physical activity and habits. These changes include the processes that occur in the pubic symphysis, the auricular facet, the sternal end of the first and fourth ribs, the sacrum, the acetabulum and, dental wear, less accurately, the closure of the cranial sutures. But in this case of disaster the pubic symphysis, and the auricular facet many times could be broken or difficult to analyze.

In order to make the expert work more effective, our own standards have been developed based on the Cuban population, to estimate parameters of the biological profile (sex, height, age and ancestral pattern). Some of these have been published in Spanish and Mexican anthropology journals. These standards have been included in computer algorithms that speed up the process of estimating the parameters. All of this has been validated in work in other provinces of the country, in air disasters with very good results, and in other countries that have a similar population or as a methodology that is useful for developing their own standards. Likewise, contributions have been made with other entities to improve the software, as occurred with FORDISC, by including Cuban samples in the latest versions.

In the same way, another group that includes psychologists and psychiatrists is in charge of obtaining antemortem information (data provided by relatives, friends, doctors, dentists, medical records, X-rays, etc.). Computerized axial tomography (CT), magnetic resonance (MRI) and DNA profiles from interviews with relatives and close friends. All that research is later corroborated with what was found in the morgue. There are models made by Interpol for the collection of both antemortem and postmortem data,

Once, the fragments or bodies have been classified, it is now possible to begin to make the absolute identification. First, you start with the extreme individuals: pilots (their topographic location in the place of discovery helps a lot), children, pregnant women, and easily detectable disabled people.

In some countries, positive identification is only considered when it is carried out using fingerprint methods, dental comparison or DNA, and this does not always have to be the case, since in an air disaster, there are often a closed number of victims. Let us give an example: a plane crashes into an uninhabited place, and all 70 people on board die; it is known that among those people, there was only one who had a hip prosthesis. In the search, the fragment or corpse with the prosthesis is found, and it is not necessary to carry out DNA studies in this case. The same occurs with other elements such as intrauterine devices, certain surgical interventions, and certain tattoos, among other elements.

In the last 25 years, more than ten disasters with multiple victims have occurred in Cuba, six of them within the national territory and two in other countries with Cuban deaths and active participation of forensic anthropologists in them. This has allowed us to accumulate experiences and work methodologies that are only achieved by participating in these disasters. Each disaster has its particularities and the positive results (identification of all the victims) will depend on the knowledge acquired in previous events.

Table 1 shows some data on recent air disasters, as well as the number of victims and the time it took to identify them, where most of the bodies were charred and fragmented. It can be observed how the work time is reduced in the latest disasters, if the number of deaths is taken into account; this has been recognized not only by the national authorities but by international entities such as the Red Cross. The participation of forensic anthropologists in this has been fundamental, although never more than two participated.

Date	Event	Aircraft	Deaths	Time to identification
03/15/2002	Fell into a lagoon	AN-2	16	20 days
11/04/2010	Fell to the ground	ATR-72	68	26 days
04/29/2017	Crashed to the mountain	An-26	8	< 72 hours
05/18/2018	Fell to the ground	Boeing 737	112	8 days
01/29/2022	Crashed to the mountain	Mi-8	5	< 48 hours

Table 1.
Data of the most recent aircraft disasters in Cuba.

5. The 883 Aerocaribbean aircraft disaster

Cuban forensic anthropologists have participated in the identification of bodies in more than 15 air disasters with multiple victims, including one of these in 2010, where 68 people died. In this case, the importance of work at the scene of the accident can be seen. The topographic location of the remains of the victims in the plane, and the subsequent forensic anthropological study were elements of great value in identifying the cadaveric remains.

On November 4, 2010, at approximately 17:42 hours, an ATR-72-212 aircraft with registration CU-T1549 belonging to Aerocaribbean S.A. crashed and caught fire near the province of Sancti Spíritus, Cuba. It had taken off from Antonio Maceo International Airport in Santiago de Cuba at 16:45 hours on the same day, bound for José Martí International Airport in Havana, killing all 68 people on board (7 crew and 61 passengers) (**Figure 1**).

After losing control of the aircraft due to icing and fracture of the tail fin, among other mishaps, the plane crashed into the ground in an isolated wooded area in the center of the country, covered with marabou (*Dichrostachys cinerea*), a thorny tree that can reach 5 meters in height, and turn the area into a very dense area.

The aircraft had accumulated more than half of the fuel for the trip, so when it hit the ground, it caught fire and burned for more than five hours without being able to be extinguished due to the difficult access to the area of the accident, due to the characteristics of the vegetation described, it was difficult for the firefighting teams. From the beginning, it was known that there were no survivors, and from the place where it crashed, the human remains corresponded only to the crew members and passengers, that is, the 68 people on board (**Figure 2**).

After the fire was extinguished, a group of specialists from the Institute of Legal Medicine led by the unfortunately recently deceased Dr. Jorge González Pérez, criminalistics and police instruction, appeared at the scene and proceeded to remove the human remains.

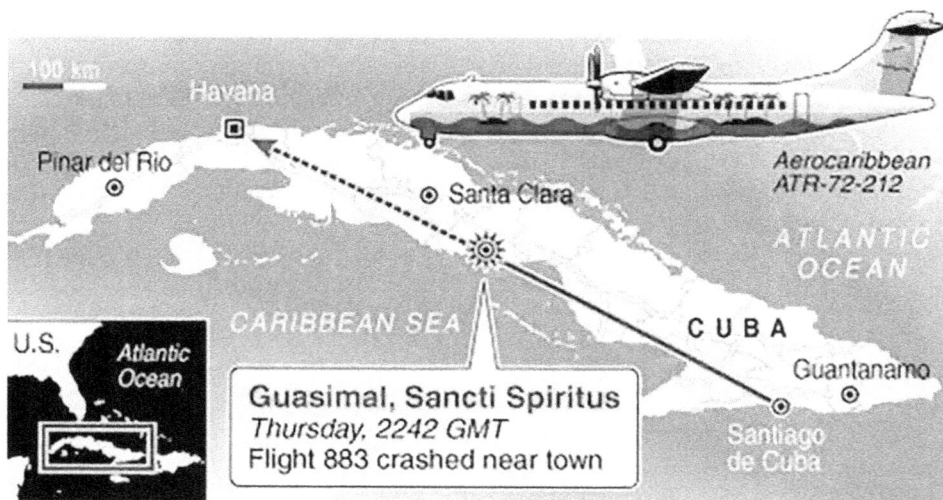

Figure 1.
Trajectory of ATR-72-212, flight 883 of Aerocaribbean (Available from: www.abc.es).

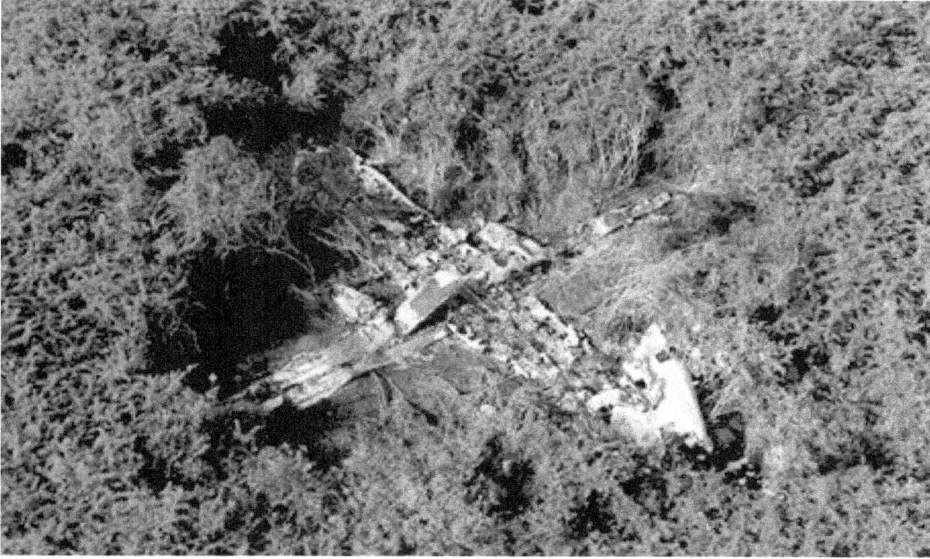

Figure 2.
The state of the plane after the impact, note the "integrity" of the plane and the lush surrounding vegetation. Screenshot from an archive video.

The plane fell completely vertically, on its belly, so there was no displacement on the ground and that allowed it to remain intact despite the subsequent fire. A measuring tape was placed in the center, in an anteroposterior direction to the tail, and the remains began to be recovered according to the metric reference. The groups of remains were noted according to the distance from the front end of the aircraft to where they were located and to the tape, on the transverse axis. (**Figure 3**).

Work at the scene of the accident should not be delayed because the hot and humid Cuban climate favors the putrefaction process and the corpses decompose quickly. The remains were stored in nylon bags, duly labeled and identified, to then be transported in a refrigerated truck to the Institute of Legal Medicine, where the identification process would be carried out.

The work of identifying the remains at the Institute of Legal Medicine.

The remains were mostly charred and very fragmented. The work teams at the morgue were made up of forensic doctors and criminal experts. Another group was in charge of collecting antemortem information and police instructions to guide everything and manage the boarding video, a very important element to know some physical characteristics, clothing, etc., of the passengers.

In these cases, forensic anthropologists are not included in the groups. The two that existed in Cuba until that time worked at the Institute of Legal Medicine itself, the then masters in sciences Héctor Soto Izquierdo and Dodany Machado Mendoza. The anthropologists are in charge of the classification process of the remains, giving the elements of the biological profile (sex, ancestral pattern, age and height) of each corpse or fragment. They must be present in all cases and are assisted by the forensic doctor and the criminal expert.

This classification process was cumbersome because some initial bags contained remains of more than one corpse and the skulls in more than 80% had not been

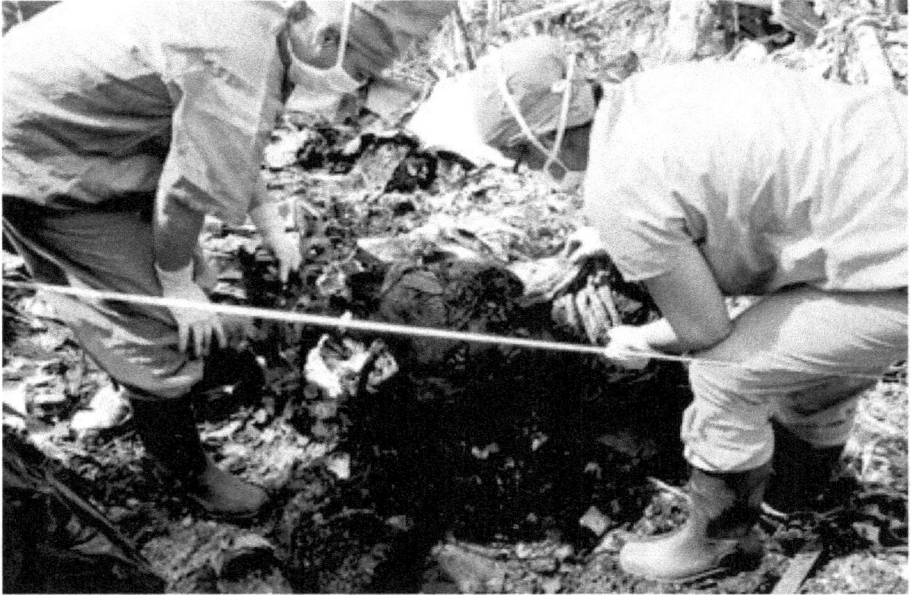

Figure 3.
Collection of the remains with reference to the measuring tape (Archive photo).

recovered since they exploded with the heat; the abdominal and leg region was what was most preserved in most cases.

Based on algorithms created to work with fragments [10–12], it was possible to determine height and sex in the most destroyed cases. The X-rays allowed us to estimate the approximate age from the fragments of the spine and ribs.

Despite all this, after eight days had passed, only six corpses had been identified, two by facial comparison (they were practically intact): the pilot and copilot, whose uniforms were well preserved and were topographically located in the front portion of the aircraft; the security guard who was carrying his gun and handcuffs and did not have serious injuries; and the 10-year-old boy who was the only minor on the plane.

The ATR-72-212 was in emergency mode for about six minutes until it fell, so the instructions should have been to sit in their seats and fasten their seatbelts. Taking this into account, the author of this chapter suggested the possibility of analyzing the topographic location of the remains, compared to the one that the passengers on the plane should have had, starting from the fact that the plane maintained its structure and the arrangement of the passengers in the seats, although they could move due to the impact, should correspond to the position referred to in the flight list.

The planes of the plane were searched and with the record of the locations in meters of the remains with respect to the central axis of the plane, a comparison could be made between who occupied the seats and how the remains appeared. Once elements of the biological profile of each corpse or fragment were known, having received the antemortem information, as well as DNA samples and dental and radiographic records of the passengers, the topographic location was assessed to whom each cadaveric portion could correspond (**Figure 4**).

For example, in row 16 on the right, there should have been a 56-year-old woman, in row 15, a young adult couple (36 and 37 years old); and in row 14 on the same side, a couple of older adults (65 and 70 years old). The layout of the location and the

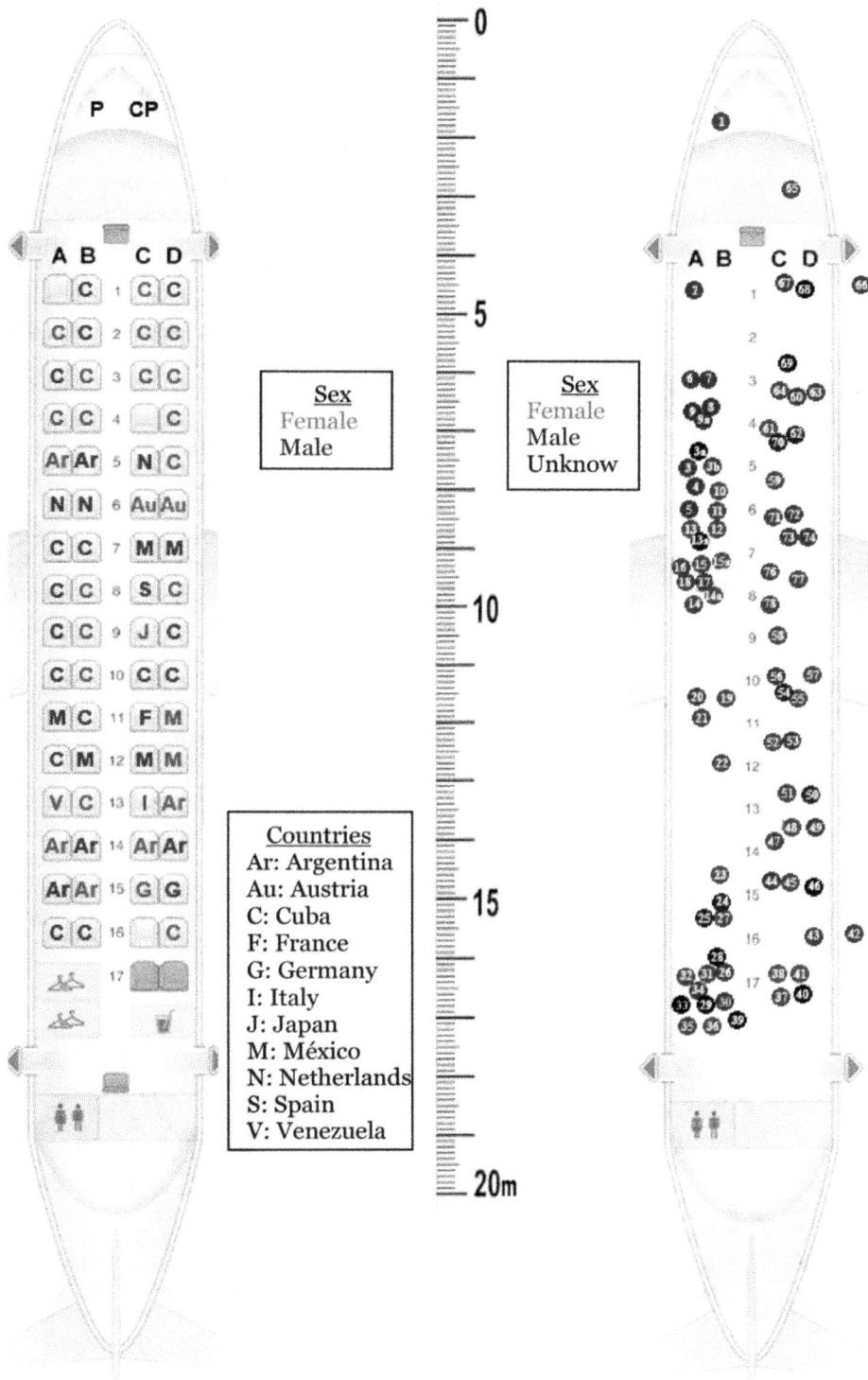

Figure 4.
Passenger seating arrangement (left) and location of groups of human remains at the scene of the accident (right).

anthropological study of the remains were reviewed, and this showed that in the last row, there were remains of a woman of about 50 to 60 years old (#41), a possible passenger, a young woman (#38) and a man (#37), who was later identified as crew members; in the penultimate row, a young woman had already been identified whose body was ejected from the aircraft on impact and was not affected by the fire (#42), and a tall man of 30 to 40 years old (#43). In the third to last row, the remains of a man (#45) and a woman (#44), aged over 60 years, were found. DNA testing confirmed the identities.

Despite the fact that there were a total of 61 passengers and 7 crew members, more than 80 groups of remains were collected due to the high fragmentation that occurred. When a body was identified, the remains closest to it were sought and the biological profile was compared with the physical characteristics of the closest passengers. In fact, there was one case where the male person (seat 3B) changed seats with a woman seat (1A), because their father was in another location and the remains of the father (#9) and daughter (#9A) appeared together.

With this information, DNA studies were carried out, focusing directly on who these remains might belong to. This was followed successively with the rest of the locations; two days later, 26 bodies had already been identified, and after another 48 hours, 39 passenger remains were already identified.

Most of the bodies were very destroyed and only a few remains remained. In fact, only the remains of seven passengers could be identified by dentistry (one of them is shown in **Figures 5** and **6**), despite having dental records for more than 20. There were two cases where only a foot was found in one and a fragment of a thigh in the other, with the peculiarity that the foot showed a metal device for the treatment of hallux valgus (**Figure 7**), and the thigh a metal hip prosthesis (head of femur) (**Figure 8**). Only two people on the plane matched these characteristics. X-rays of the first case were available and a comparison was made. The second was the only passenger with a hip prosthesis, so they were declared identified without difficulties.

Surgically implanted devices have become increasingly common, so knowledge of their variety, utility, manufacturer, and how to use identification numbers can assist in the identification process [2].

In the wing area, where the fuel is stored, the fuel ignited on impact, causing explosions and the bodies were destroyed to a large extent, with the passengers in these seats being the ones whose identification took the longest.

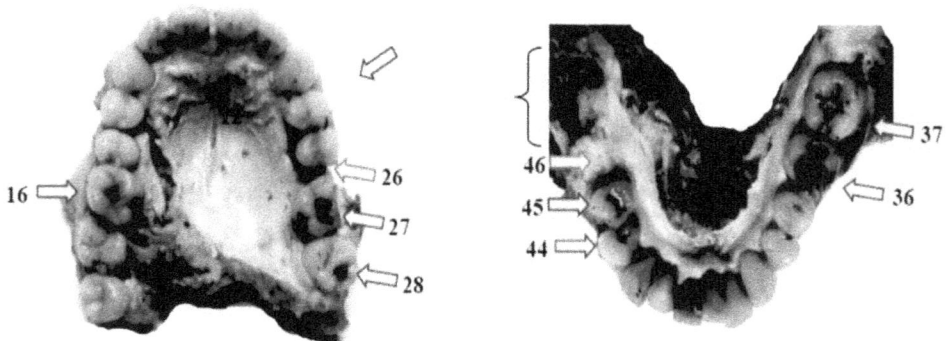

Figure 5.
Dental arches corresponding to the investigated skull of #38, with blue arrows indicating the filled teeth (16, 26, 27, 28, 36, 37, 44 and 45). Note the spaces (red arrows) resulting from antemortem extractions and the missing arch fragment (black key) (photos taken by the author).

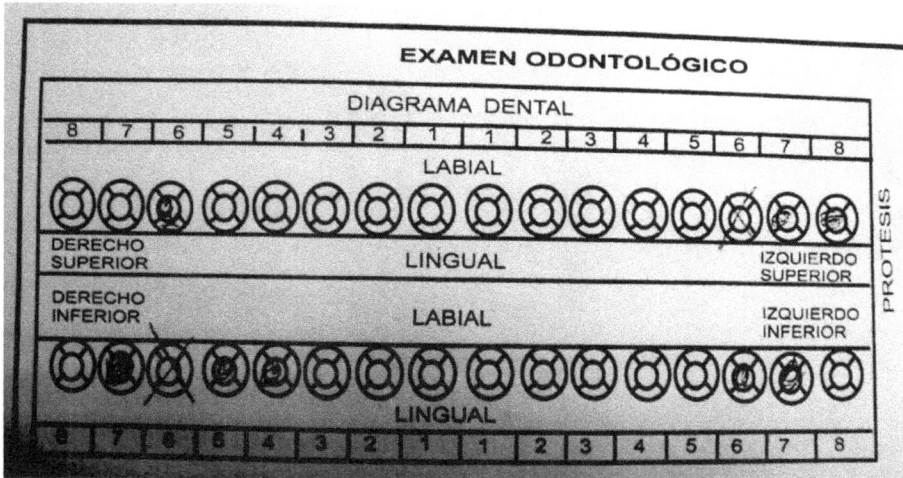

Figure 6.
Photocopy of the dental chart performed on citizen A in September 2010 (the markings in the original were in blue). The coincidences with the elements found in the oral autopsy of #38 are noted. Photo taken by the author.

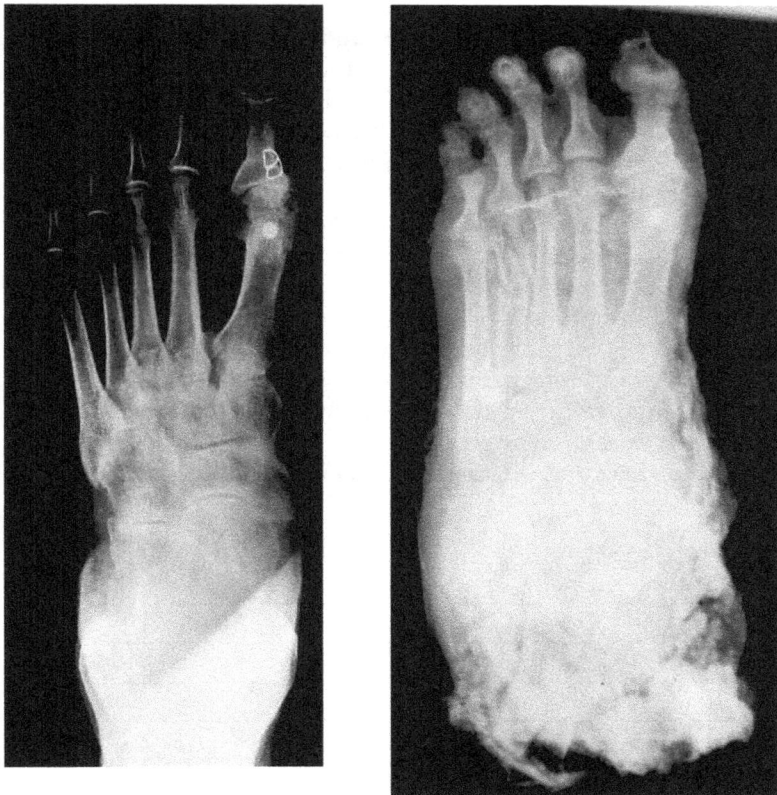

Figure 7.
Antemortem radiograph (left) of the patient's left foot showing the metal device for the treatment of hallux valgus, *compared with the postmortem radiograph (right) of the patient's left foot, which showed a similar device. Photos taken by the author.*

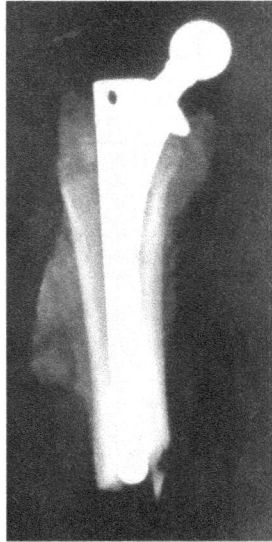

Figure 8.
Fragment of thigh found with metal hip prosthesis and showing the soft tissue attached. Photo taken by the author.

After 20 days of hard work, all passengers and crew were identified, although in some cases, only small fragments remained. It is worth noting that identification is done by consensus, all the postmortem information collected and compared with the antemortem data is taken to a meeting where, if all those present (more than 20 people including forensic experts, anthropologists and experts) agree with what was presented, the body or part of it is identified and the police instruction informs the relatives so that they can present themselves and explain how the identification was reached. **Table 2** shows the most important methods for identifying the remains.

It should be noted that in all cases, the forensic topography was highly indicative, as well as the classification work carried out by the forensic anthropologists which helped to determine who each of the remains studied might belong to.

This case showed that organization and teamwork are essential. Good work at the scene of the accident, together with experience in handling fragmented and charred corpses, facilitated the achievement of the result. The work during those days of identification was exhausting, seeking precision in all the details because in some

Identification methods	Victims
DNA	54
Odontology	7
Clothing and belongings (crew)	3
Osteosynthesis material	2
Facial comparison	2
Total	68

Table 2.
Main identification methods used on the 68 passengers and crew of the ATR 72–212.

cases there was little available. Many X-rays were taken and all possible methods were applied to speed up the work.

It also taught us how important rest is; the first 10 days, we worked with little time to sleep, and this had an impact on the work, an aspect that was taken into account in subsequent disasters and the results were much more satisfactory.

6. Conclusions

Forensic Anthropology shows a conscientious scientific work with a high social and humanitarian content. It uses specific knowledge and experience adquired to assist in the administration of justice, and important work in disaster victim identification, to find the remains and expedite the process of identifying corpses and other issues in the interest of the relatives.

The mission of the forensic anthropologist in multiple-victim events is not only focused on determining the biological profile but is also linked to the rest of the investigation phases, where the importance of their integration into the remains recovery teams is highlighted, as well as in the classification of the remains in the morgue. It is in these two areas where the work of these professionals can bring more benefits.

Good management in the diligence of removing the remains or parts of corpses will optimize subsequent work and speed up the identification of the corpses. Although most international standards in the field of major catastrophes recognize the figure of the forensic anthropologist, their intervention cannot be said to be widespread. The experience gathered in events where anthropologists have intervened demonstrates their potential, by simplifying tasks and facilitating the process of identifying human remains, with the speed in obtaining results and the considerable reduction in the number of genetic analyses, with the consequent economic savings that this entails. This work is not only the responsibility of anthropologists; the functioning of a work team that includes specialists from all branches of forensic sciences makes it easier to obtain the desired results with the best quality and professionalism in the shortest time possible.

Acknowledgements

With this work, we would like to honor the memory of two eminent forensic experts, Dr. Jorge González Pérez (1952–2024), medical examiner and disaster expert, and M.Sc. Héctor Soto Izquierdo (1949–2022), a Forensic Anthropologist for 47 years, who actively participated in a large number of catastrophes.

A special thanks to all the staff of the Institute of Legal Medicine and the rest of Cuban specialists of forensic sciences for their dedicated work when these types of events occur.

Author details

Dodany Machado Mendoza
Forensic Anthropologist of the Institute of Legal Medicine, Havana, Cuba

*Address all correspondence to: dodany@gmail.com

IntechOpen

References

[1] Burns KR. Manual de Antropología Forense. 1st ed. Bellaterra: Barcelona; 2007. p. 446

[2] Barbería Marcalain E. Catástrofes. Identificación de víctimas y otros aspectos médico-forenses. 1st ed. Barcelona: Elsevier; 2015. p. 553

[3] Vallejo G, Alonso A. La identificación genética en grandes catástrofes: avances científicos y normativos en España. Revista Española de Medicina Legal. 2009;**2009**(35):19-27

[4] Busuttil A, Jones JSP, Green MA. Deaths in Major Disasters – The pathologist's Role. 2nd ed. London: The Royal College of Pathologists; 2000

[5] Williams JAY, Weedn VW. Disaster Victim Identification in the 21st Century. AUS Perspective. Chichester, UK: Wiley & Sons LTD; 2021. p. 553

[6] PAHO. Marco de respuesta a emergencias. Washington DC: Organización Mundial de la Salud; 2013. Available from: http://www.who.int/hac/about/erf/es/

[7] Wisner B, Adams J. Environmental Health in Emergencies and Disasters: A Practical Guide. Ginebra: Organización Mundial de la Salud; 2002

[8] Arcos González P, Castro Delgado R, Cuartas Álvarez T, Pérez-Berrocal Alonso J. Terrorismo, salud pública y sistemas sanitarios. Revista Española de Salud Pública. 2009;**83**:361-370

[9] International Committee of the Red Cross. Guía Práctica para la recuperación y análisis de restos humanos en contextos de violaciones a los Derechos Humanos

e infracciones contra el Derecho Internacional Humanitario. Lima, Perú: Ministerio Público de la Nación; 2017. p. 48

[10] Machado D, Garcell F, Pérez V. Estimación del sexo a partir del fémur mediante funciones discriminantes, en cubanos de ascendencia hispánica. Revista Internacional de Antropología y Odontología Forense. 2021;**4**(3):6-14

[11] Machado DY, Pérez V. Estimación del sexo por las epífisis del radio en una muestra de cubanos. Anales de Antropología UNAM. 2022;**56**(2):13-20

[12] Machado D, Urgellés LA, Pérez V. Estimación de la longitud del húmero a partir de sus epífisis y asociación de fragmentos proximales con distales, en cubanos de ascendencia hispánica. Revista Internacional de Antropología y Odontología Forense. 2024;**7**(2):26-36

Chapter 6

Recent Advances in Medical Ethics

Praveen Kumar Pradhan

Abstract

This chapter delves into the evolving landscape of medical ethics, addressing the challenges brought forth by rapid technological advancements, changes in societal values, and the globalization of healthcare. It explores key developments such as the ethical implications of artificial intelligence in medicine, personalized medicine, genetic engineering, and end-of-life care. By examining case studies and real-world scenarios, this chapter highlights how ethical frameworks are being redefined to accommodate novel healthcare practices, ensuring patient autonomy, equity, and transparency. It also discusses the role of ethics committees, regulatory bodies, and legal systems in adapting to these changes while safeguarding public trust in medical practice.

Keywords: ethics, autonomy, privacy, AI, dignity, rights, confidentiality, bias, technology, recent advances

1. Introduction

The modern healthcare system is directed by medical ethics, which are the well-discussed principles of right and wrong. Medical ethics assures us that the practice of medicine is not just a matter of decisions made in the doctor's office but is also a matter of societal values, cultural norms, justice, and the welfare of the patient. Navigating the healthcare system and making decisions within it seems to be only getting more complex, even as it gets more high-tech. At the same time, there seem to be just as many opportunities, if not more, for medical practitioners to make unethical decisions.

Medical ethics centres on four key principles. They are:

a. Autonomy: Respect the rights of patients to make their own healthcare decisions.

b. Beneficence: Promote the well-being of our patients and act in their best interests.

c. Non-maleficence: Avoid causing harm and see to it that our interventions do not result in needless suffering.

d. Justice: Ensure fairness and see to it that all persons have at least an equal opportunity to receive humanity and respect those rights, too.

These principles serve as the moral compass for healthcare providers and help us solve disputes. A situation might arise where a doctor's ethics could be put to the test. A patient could flatly refuse a treatment that the physician knows could be life-saving. The patient's reasons for doing so might be based on core beliefs or values that the patient holds dear. This could make for a very delicate situation indeed. The physician has to balance beneficence, doing what is in the best interest of the patient, and non-maleficence, ensuring no harm comes to the patient. They also have to respect the patient's autonomy. Medical ethics extends quite a bit beyond individual cases. These inquiries emphasize the evolving character of medical ethics. Medical ethics must not only keep pace with the advancements of modern medicine but also adapt to medicine's changing societal expectations and new ethical conundrums.

2. Historical development of medical ethics

This follows the line of thought that there have always been medical ethics and it was not solely confined to Western civilization. A better comprehension of medicine, of mankind, and of ethics began with the ancient societies and developed further into the modern era defining moments.

2.1 Ancient foundations

When patients were looked after, the healers had ethical obligations, and this can be traced back to ancient Egypt, India, China and Greece.

- Ancient Egypt: The Ebers Papyrus (circa 1550 BCE) is the oldest medical literature available; it at least provides treatments for different diseases and shows that there was some form of code of ethics that was expected of its practitioners. Practitioners were regarded as representatives of the gods and hence were required to practice within acceptable moral standards [1].

- Ancient India: The Charaka Samhita (around first century BCE), a working Ayurveda text speaks more about the physician's own self and his morality. It was required that the breast doctor was merciful, trustful and self-interested in the patient, masked right to treat, which ruled out harming actions towards patients than those already afflicted with injuries or illness [2].

- Ancient China: With the influence of both Confucianism and Taoism, Chinese medicine supplemented the practice with an ethical component. The preaching of Confucius stressed harmony, respect towards life, and the duty of the doctor to society. Taoism also placed importance on the physical and the spiritual but promoted a more balanced view towards health [2].

2.2 The Hippocratic oath

The Hippocratic Oath is a medical pledge that originated in Ancient Greece in the fifth century BCE. Hippocrates is known as the father of medicine. This oath sets out the basic ethical principles that are relevant today. The doctors vowed to keep things secret about patients' information. The first commitment not to harm is one of non-maleficence, explicitly stated "I will not intentionally do harm related medical advice and treatment". The oath states that the health and well-being of patients must always come before one's self or financial gain [1].

The Hippocratic Oath established a standard of conduct by which physicians should live. It suggests that medicine is a moral enterprise. Doctors around the world, in a variety of forms, continue to take this vow to this day.

2.3 The medieval times

During the medieval era, religious codes governed the medical field. The guidance of various religions helped health service providers.

- In Europe, Christians thought that taking care of the sick was a moral duty. Hospitals established by monasteries became instruments of healing and comfort to the sick. Ethical principles such as charity, humility and the sanctity of life were of utmost importance [3].

- During the Islamic Golden Age, physicians and physicians began to advance medical ethics. The Canon of Medicine, which he wrote, gave a set of instructions for the doctor so that he will respect life and be compassionate. Also, it states about integrity in the use of medicines.

Asian medical traditions integrate spirituality with ethics in Buddhism and Hinduism. Decisions were influenced by principles like ahimsa (non-violence), so treatments were in accordance with those values and were harmless [2].

2.4 The enlightenment and secular ethics

In the eighteenth and nineteenth centuries, the Enlightenment caused people to believe in reason, the right to choose, and the ability to investigate. Hence, they created medical ethics that were not based on religion. Immanuel Kant and other thinkers introduced a view of ethics called deontological ethical theory, which focuses on the physician's moral duty. In utilitarian ethical theories advocated by John Stuart Mill, decisions must be made based on the consequences that will best promote the overall good. The period also saw a professionalization of medicine. In 1847, the American Medical Association (AMA) released their first Code of Medical Ethics which pertained to confidentiality, informed consent and the medical profession [4].

2.5 The modern era: Bioethics and beyond

The twentieth century brought transformative changes to medical ethics, spurred by scientific advancements, societal shifts, and historical events. Post-World War II: Medical experiments during the Holocaust pertaining to the Nuremberg Trials where these trials exposed the revelation that these Nuremberg Trials succeeded in marking some of the renowned Nuremberg Code (1947) which is a landmark document which ensures informed consent and also resists the protection of subjects of research.

In the 1970s, the advent of bioethics enhanced the field of medical ethics by adding such things as genetic engineering, organ transplantation and reproductive technologies. The respect, beneficence and justice with respect to human research principles were supplied to the Belmont Report in 1979 [5].

Questions were raised about questions of autonomy, what constitutes death and the extent of advance directives that would mitigate the relatives' exposure to what was perceived as an impending tortious behavior in landmark cases like Karen Ann Quinlan (1976) and Terri Schiavo (2005).

2.6 Contemporary ethical challenges

In the twenty-first century, medical ethics faces unprecedented challenges. Concerns on AI healthcare integration are in the form of algorithmic bias, transparency, accountability. These technologies are needed to have equitable and trustworthy use and ethical frameworks to ensure them. Finally, technology have advanced to the point where there are ethical questions about "designer babies", germline modifications, and the cost of expensive therapies have evolved in genomic medicine and CRISPR [6]. During the COVID-19 pandemic vaccine distribution revealed and created new ethical challenges in regards to balancing individual rights to public health measures [7].

3. Medicine: Recent developments in medical ethics

It is an AI integration into medicine that is a paradigm of a new approach to how healthcare is set up, researched, and delivered. The power of the algorithms and vast datasets have given it the impetus to make possible immense progress in diagnostics, treatment personalization and healthcare accessibility. However, these opportunities pose ethical challenges to the current practice and prospects of health care. This essay discusses the major transformative applications of AI, the ethical issues arising therefrom, and how to handle these issues.

3.1 Applications of artificial intelligence in medicine

AI's role in healthcare spans a wide array of applications, each contributing to improved efficiency, accuracy and patient outcomes.

3.1.1 Personalized and precision medicine

Precision medicine requires analysis of complex patient data such as genetic profiles to tailor treatments to an individual's specific needs, a job that AI can handle. AI models also suggest, in oncology, the response of a tumor to specific drugs in order to help oncologists to decide which treatment plans are more effective [8].

Thus, pharmacogenomics [8] defines AI to identify how a patient's genetic makeup may affect drug metabolism so as to reduce its adverse effects and optimize therapeutic results. It has revolutionized diagnostics by improving accuracy and reducing time-to-diagnosis. For instance, deep learning algorithms are used in medical imaging to identify abnormalities such as tumors, fractures, and vascular conditions.

Now, diagnostic tools powered by AI, read through imaging data (e.g., CT scans and MRIs) exceptionally accurately. For example, these tools, like Aidoc for radiology and PathAI for histopathology, help reduce how long clinicians take to detect abnormalities [9]. In personalized medicine, AI diagnostics help each patient get personalized diagnostic insights and do not offer services that the patient does not need.

3.1.2 Surgical assistance

AI-enhanced robotic systems have altered surgical procedures. Tools like Da Vinci Surgical System tools provide unmatched precision for minimally invasive surgery, making recovery periods shorter, enhancing patient outcomes, and reducing recovery times. These systems are guided by AI algorithms to ability these systems to guide the surgeons in navigating the complex anatomy [10].

3.1.3 Drug discovery

Integration of AI in pharmacology has had a huge effect on the way drugs are found. AI algorithms search molecular databases and suggest families of drugs that may be the most promising drug candidates, predict their interaction with specific genetic profiles, and to optimize the design of clinical trials. The advances of these technologies also benefit personalized medicine as the drugs are tailored towards genetic subpopulations, achieving higher efficacy and decreased side effects. For instance, the deep learning of molecular interactions to accelerate the identification of personalized therapeutic targets is accomplished through AI-driven platforms such as Atomwise [11].

3.1.4 Predictive analytics and public health

Predictive tools powered by AI can predict disease outbreaks, predict hospital admission trends and predict patient deterioration. For example, AI systems incorporate EHRs to predict heart attack injuries, thereby allowing timely interventions [12]. During the COVID-19 pandemic, AI models in epidemiology monitor disease spread as tools to predict hotspots and guide containment strategies [13]. By analyzing patient data alongside clinical guidelines and translating this into individualized treatment regimens that cannot be replicated by humans. AI systems like IBM Watson for Oncology (that evaluates treatment options with regeneration of the tumor genetics and patient preferences, precision care is developed for cancer patients) [14]. The foundational science of personalized medicine, genomics, has progressed rapidly thanks to AI. Machine learning algorithms analyze massive genomic datasets to:

- Identify genetic mutations: CRISPR-based prediction models can identify specific mutations that can be associated with inherited diseases or cancer risks [15].

- Interpret gene expression: Gene expression data can be analyzed using algorithms to predict disease susceptibility and to subsequently guide treatment strategies [16].

- Integrate multi-omic data: Together, these data can be used by AI to bring a holistic view of a patient's biological profile from genomics, proteomics, metabolomics and microbiomics [17].

For illustration, AI-oriented tools like Google Deep Variant, have increased the accuracy of identifying genetic variations to a far better extent, leading to early diagnosis and targeted interventions [18]. Predictive analytics is the domain of AI, using patient data to predict when and how the disease will progress. AI systems analyze patterns of health records, imaging data, and lifestyle metrics to detect early signs of chronic conditions linked with diabetes, cardiovascular diseases and cancer. Predictions based on this early intervention can significantly improve outcomes [19].

3.1.5 Virtual health assistants and telemedicine

AI chatbots and virtual assistants help patients by taking care of symptom checks, booking appointments and reminding them about medicine. These tools extend medical practice to areas with limited resources and relieve the strain on medical professionals [13].

4. Genetic engineering: Recent developments in medical ethics

The intersection of artificial intelligence (AI) and genetic engineering represents one of the most groundbreaking areas of modern science. As AI tools become more sophisticated, they have enabled deeper insights into genetic research, opened new avenues for gene editing, and significantly advanced personalized medicine. However, with these advancements come substantial ethical dilemmas and concerns regarding their responsible use. From personalized gene therapy to the potential for "designer babies", the integration of AI in genetic engineering requires careful ethical scrutiny, particularly as it influences societal structures, cultural norms, and the very essence of human genetics.

4.1 AI's role in advancing genetic engineering

4.1.1 Genomic analysis and Interpretation

One of the most important gifts AI has given to genetic engineering is its capability to manage and process large amounts of genetic data. The analysis of genomic data with traditional methods was very tedious and needed lots of human expertise. However, the revolution of this process has been facilitated by AI, through machine learning algorithms that gave new speed and accuracy in interpreting complex genetic information. Genetic data can be sifted by machine learning algorithms to find patterns that indicate how genetic diseases manifest themselves. For example, in 2013, AI was used to detect SNPs linked to Alzheimer's and cardiovascular diseases, which then facilitated the prediction of disease susceptibility and individualizing treatment methods [20]. Large-scale datasets can be used to analyze how genetic variations affect health outcomes and predict how an AI-based model will predict the outcomes. The ability to predict is fundamental to the development of personalized therapies based on an individual's genetic profile [21]. However, genomic data is often combined with other types of omic data, such as transcriptomic, proteomic and metabolomic, to provide a more complete set of information on a person's health. Integration and analysis of these multi-dimensional datasets becomes doable in the presence of AI, and provides new insights into novel biomarkers and gene-environment interactions [22]. Genetic engineering, overpowered by AI's computational power, has started to develop towards a more systematic and holistic approach to human gene analytics (in disease prevention and treatment).

4.1.2 Precision gene editing: Enhancing CRISPR and beyond

One of the most disruptive genetic engineering technologies is gene editing, namely CRISPR Cas9. CRISPR can be used to make precise changes to the genetic code to repair genetic disorders, change agricultural traits and even open up the door to study features of biology that were unimaginable before. AI plays an essential role in optimizing gene-editing processes. While gene editing technologies like CRISPR are powerful, one of the challenges is that the changes that are made to the DNA must be accurate and not cause unintentional genetic mutations elsewhere in the genome. However, AI systems can assess huge genetic datasets to determine where possible "off target" effects could occur, enabling gene editing tools to be more accurate [23]. Guide RNAs guide the Cas9 enzyme to certain locations within the genome, and this localization is critical to use of CRISPR technology. To design these guide RNAs and tune their efficiency AI tools like deep learning algorithms are used [24]. Precise genome editing especially for human clinical trials has relied increasingly on the AI-driven design of guide RNAs. AI tools simulate the effects of particular genetic modifications before actually doing the gene editing. Through combining this simulation process with high-performance computing, researchers can now predict the phenotypic effects of gene edits, speeding up and reducing the need for time consuming and expensive *in vivo* trials [25]. As gene editing technologies move towards precision medicine, made humanly possible by AI, there is the hope of treatment for many once incurable conditions.

4.1.3 Gene therapy and AI in drug discovery

One of the most exciting uses of genetic engineering is as a gene therapy to correct, inactivate or replace defective genes and treat or cure diseases. As AI has improved the design of therapeutic strategies, better delivery mechanisms and predicted outcomes from potential gene therapies, it has accelerated the development of gene therapies. Key ways in which AI supports gene therapy include Target Identification, Optimizing Gene Delivery and Personalized Gene Therapy. Genomic data can be sifted through by AI algorithms and novel druggable targets are found. By studying genetic pathways and mutations, AI models can help by identifying which genes or proteins are most likely to be good, targeted gene therapy therapeutic targets [26]. The problem with gene therapy is to be able to ensure that the modified genetic material gets to the right place. AI helps in identifying the most ideal delivery mechanisms that can be viral vectors or non-viral methods, but the gene therapy should reach the cells that require that [27]. Because genetic diversity is an underlying factor in how people respond to medical treatments, AI is at the pedestal of personalizing gene therapies. This can be used to tailor therapies to individual patients and better enable effectiveness while reducing the risk of adverse effects [28]. The future of gene therapy is bright, considering that drug discovery processes can now be done faster and more accurately with AI, and especially for genetic disorders such as muscular dystrophy, cystic fibrosis, and inherited retinal diseases is a tantalizing prospect.

4.1.4 Synthetic biology and AI-driven genome design

Synthetic biology involves creating organisms with customized genetic materials that may not occur naturally. The use of AI in synthetic biology allows scientists to engineer microbial cells, plants, and animals with novel properties, thus pushing the boundaries of what genetic engineering can achieve.

AI plays an indispensable role in synthetic biology through Gene Synthesis, Whole Genome Synthesis and Environmental Adaptability. AI systems optimize the design of synthetic genes, predicting how newly designed genetic sequences will behave within living organisms. AI algorithms can suggest modifications to genetic sequences to optimize expression and functionality, enabling the creation of engineered organisms that produce biofuels, pharmaceuticals, or agricultural products [29]. In synthetic biology, AI enables the design of entire genomes for organisms with tailored capabilities, such as algae engineered to produce biofuels or bacteria designed to clean up environmental pollutants. AI helps to model and predict how these synthetic organisms will behave in natural ecosystems, addressing ecological concerns and reducing risks [30]. AI models help predict how synthetic organisms will interact with their environments, optimizing their stability, resistance to disease, and other traits critical for their success in real-world applications [31]. In agriculture, AI-driven synthetic biology has already led to the creation of genetically modified crops with increased resistance to pests, better nutritional content, and enhanced resilience to climate change.

5. Ethical implications of AI in medicine and genetic engineering

While AI has introduced remarkable advancements, its implementation raises several ethical issues that require careful consideration:

5.1 Transparency and explainability

In particular "deep learning" based AI algorithms suffer from often being the so called "black box" failing to provide the decisions they provide in a way that is easy to interpret. AI generated recommendations might not get healthcare providers on board without the explanations. Simply, they may be reluctant to accept diagnoses or treatments from opaque systems [32]. Integrating AI into the clinical workflow is problematic because it lacks explainability, in addition to the fact that the rationale for AI decisions differs from human judgement [32]. Building trust and enabling informed decision-making via the development of interpretable AI models, including decision tree or rule-based systems [32]. So many AI systems "do what they do", you do not really have an idea what is going on. This lack of transparency can undermine trust in AI-driven healthcare. Informed Consent and Autonomy Obtaining informed consent for AI-driven interventions is complex, as patients may not fully understand how AI algorithm's function [17]. Efficient communication and education of the patient are important so that important ethical decisions may be made. If Patients cannot understand the rationale behind the AI recommendation, they may avoid accepting it. It is important for clinicians to understand AI outputs to trust the systems and make informed decisions. Explaining AI (XAI) advances seek to make algorithms better interpretable, and in turn more trusted and accountable.

5.2 Bias

Like other AI systems, the biases in the data used to train a pipeline are often reflected in the results. These biases can lead to unequal treatment outcomes. For example, AI tools used in dermatology, studies have revealed, perform worse for darker skin tones as training datasets most commonly consist of images of lighter skin. Because of such disadvantaged communities, biased AI systems are at risk of aggravating existing inequalities [33]. Biases are mitigated if we create diverse and representative datasets coupled with rigorous testing and validation [33]. The amount of data that we are training our AI models on can only be as biased as they are. Many datasets lack diversity, leading to Underrepresentation and Health Disparities. With the underrepresentation of minority populations in training data, the prediction may be less accurate for minority populations [34]. Recent studies suggest that operating biased algorithms can worsen existing inequity in access to quality care in under-served communities and groups [35].

One example is that a study discovered that an AI model that predicted health risks allocated fewer assets to black sufferers than to white sufferers (despite advanced need) [19]. To solve this, we need several datasets and an ongoing auditing of AI models. Genetic data is one of the most sensitive types of personal information, and its use in AI-driven genetic engineering raises significant privacy concerns. But there is potential for genetic discrimination if employers or insurers can get a hold of people's genetic information. For instance, reproductive decisions may be prohibited on the basis of genetic predispositions to particular genetic disorders [36]. With every genetic data being collected and stored, the risk of data breaches is increasing. Genetic data, if turned loose, can be used maliciously with devastating consequences to the individual and the family [37]. While genetic research using AI necessitates huge data sets, much of it is already being produced. Participation in genetic studies should be assured from individuals by obtaining informed consent. In some cases, the complexity of AI models stymies people's ability to understand how their data is going to be used, which calls into question transparency and consent [38]. The ethical frameworks about genetic data must protect individuals' genetic data and strictly restrict privacy, data sharing, and consent.

5.3 Privacy and data security

The reliance on AI on extensive patient data raises significant concerns about privacy and data security. Data probably is not collected just in isolation when patients share it with third parties to help build an AI model [39]. Health systems can be compromised by cyberattacks, and such cyberattacks can compromise sensitive patient information, undermining trust [39]. The General Data Protection Regulation (GDPR) is crucial to protecting patient privacy in order to comply with standards like this. The deployment of ethical AI includes encryption, anonymization, and best-in-class cybersecurity [39]. Data such as genetic sequences, health records and lifestyle information are sentimental data that are heavily relied on for personalized medicine. The collection, storage, and analysis of such data raise significant privacy concerns. Genetic information can be misused in terms of discrimination in employment or insurance [35]. It is also very important that patients grasp how their data will be utilized and the risks. Therefore, robust frameworks like GDPR talk of data minimization, consent and encryption [11]. Genetic data is one of the most sensitive types of personal information, and its use in AI-driven genetic engineering raises significant privacy concerns. If employers or insurers can access individuals' genetic information, then there is new potential for such discrimination. For instance, reproductive decisions may be prohibited on the basis of genetic predispositions to particular genetic disorders [36]. With every genetic data being collected and stored, the risk of data breaches is increasing. Exposure to genetic data can be exploited maliciously and cause irreversible injury to individuals and families [37]. While genetic research using AI necessitates huge data sets, much of it is already being produced. Participation in genetic studies should be assured by individuals by obtaining informed consent. Frequently, the intricacy of the AI models may leave people to wonder how exactly will their data be used and thereby raises concerns about transparency and consent [38]. Privacy and data sharing need to establish strict guidelines while protecting individual's genetic data and should mandate ethical frameworks for it.

5.4 Autonomy and human oversight

AI systems challenge traditional notions of autonomy in healthcare. AI tools recommend particular treatments and at times they coerce patients to go with what they suggest, regardless of what resonates with personal values and preferences [40]. The reliance on AI may oversee the diminishing of the physician-patient relationship as empathy and individualized care lose to the terror of the machine [40]. AI should be seen as a support to human decision-making, maintaining the human-centred nature of medicine [40]. Genetic data is one of the most sensitive types of personal information, and its use in AI-driven genetic engineering raises significant privacy concerns. The data sharing, privacy, and consent policy should be upheld while managing the use of people's genetic information.

5.5 Accountability and liability

Determining responsibility in cases of AI failure is a complex ethical and legal issue. Who is responsible for the failure in AI results: the AI developers, the healthcare providers using it, or the implementing institution? [41]. For example, current legal systems do not have clear rules regarding how to address AI-related medical errors, so new rules are needed [41].

5.6 Equity and access

AI-powered personalized medicine is often resource-intensive, raising concerns about equitable access. Low-income populations cannot potentially afford the prohibitive cost of advanced AI tools and genomic testing [35]. Due to the infrastructure required to implement AI-based healthcare solutions [42], rural or low-resource areas may lack the infrastructure to do so. To overcome these challenges, these include funding public progress towards AI healthcare and the creation of low-cost AI models. Expensive and often unaffordable, advanced AI-powered genetic interventions are out of reach for a huge majority of people on the planet. And these could even exacerbate the differences in health for people and nations, with the only ones benefiting from these advancements being the wealthy [43]. AI-driven genetic treatments are beyond reach for the low-income countries lacking infrastructure and resources to get to it. The disparity brings into question the notion of global justice, in the light of genetic engineering come to be seen as central to the modern practice of personalized medicine [44]. Consequently, deep and rich variations of genomic and evolutionary mind codes could be monopolized by large corporations, only enriching their reserves of power and resources in their hands. That could lead to a new form of genetic elitism, where only the people with substantial means can afford the genetic treatments or enhancements that will save their life [45]. To tackle these problems, authorities and global health organizations must enrich genetic engineering technologies insofar as they will remain fully fraught, regardless of socioeconomic status or geographic location.

5.7 Germline editing and "designer babies"

Genetic data is one of the most sensitive types of personal information, and its use in AI-driven genetic engineering raises significant privacy concerns. The genetic discrimination potential exists because employers or insurers could learn about an individual's genetic information. With every genetic data being collected and stored the risk of data breaches is increasing. Fortunately, genetic data must be kept securely, which could be used maliciously and harm individuals and their families [37]. While genetic research using AI necessitates huge data sets, much of it is already being produced. Participation in genetic studies should be assured from individuals by obtaining informed consent. Sometimes, the complexity of AI models complicates determining how the data of users will be used, raising questions of transparency and consent [38]. A careful balance of communication needs to be achieved to satisfy the privacy and data sharing requirements of genetic data and to maintain the integrity of personal genetic information and thus the protection of the individual.

5.8 Addressing ethical challenges

To navigate the ethical challenges of AI in medicine, several proactive measures are necessary:

a. Developing ethical guidelines: It must reintroduce AI development and application with innovative frameworks of fairness, accountability and patient rights to be governed adequately by institutions.

b. Interdisciplinary collaboration: A well-rounded solution to a complex ethical dilemma needs to engage ethicists, technologists, healthcare providers and policymakers.

c. Education and training: Training of medical practitioners in using AI technologies would allow them to assess critically the output of AI and taking informed decision.

By discussing AI in Healthcare with patients and the public, we gain trust and align with values as evidenced by the application of AI.

6. Artificial intelligence in end-of-life care and it is ethical implications

End-of-life care (EOL) is a critical aspect of healthcare that involves supporting individuals in their final days or weeks, focusing on comfort and dignity, and minimizing suffering. With advancements in medical technology, artificial intelligence (AI) is making significant strides in enhancing EOL care. AI-driven tools are helping clinicians manage complex symptoms, predict outcomes, and provide personalized care tailored to the specific needs of patients. However, the integration of AI in end-of-life care brings with it profound ethical questions. These concerns include issues of patient autonomy, decision-making, and the potential for AI to replace human compassion in the dying process. This essay explores the role of AI in end-of-life care and examines the ethical implications that arise when these technologies are employed in such sensitive and complex situations.

6.1 The role of artificial intelligence in end-of-life care

AI has found numerous applications in end-of-life care, from predictive analytics that assist in prognosis to automated systems that help manage pain and distress. AI algorithms can analyze large datasets, including medical records, to predict the likely course of a patient's illness, providing valuable insights into when a patient may be nearing the end of their life. For example, machine learning algorithms can assist in predicting when a terminally ill patient might require palliative care or when interventions, such as ventilators, may no longer be beneficial [46].

AI can also improve the management of symptoms such as pain, nausea, and anxiety, which are common in terminally ill patients. AI-enabled systems can track and analyze real-time data from wearable devices, such as heart rate, oxygen levels, and movement, to optimize the administration of medications and other therapies [47]. Additionally, AI can play a role in coordinating care, ensuring that family members, caregivers, and healthcare providers are all on the same page regarding treatment goals and patient needs.

Further, AI-based robots or virtual assistants can provide emotional support to patients who may feel isolated in their final days. AI systems can offer companionship and a sense of presence, which may be especially beneficial in environments where human interaction is limited, such as in ICU units or during the COVID-19 pandemic [48]. These technologies can engage patients in conversations, help alleviate loneliness, and offer a semblance of human interaction, even if it is not from a human being.

6.2 Ethical implications of AI in end-of-life care

First of all, the present paper identifies four major ethical concerns that arise from the integration of AI in end-of-life care, namely patient's self-governance, decision-making, and quality of care. Despite the gains that are possible by applying AI in improving clinical decision-making it is important that application of this technology does not marginalize the patient preferences and patient's self-determination.

6.3 Patient autonomy and consent

Patient autonomy—the right of patients to decide for themselves what should be done for them is among the first and foremost ethical concerns in end-of-life care. The concern is that if AI is involved in this process, patients will not fully comprehend how it works, nor will patients know the impact of them. The decision-making of AI algorithms is often black box systems, that is, their reasoning is not transparent and can often be not easily understood by patients or even by healthcare providers [49]. The lack of transparency, however, created an issue of informed consent. In practice, patients are forced to trust AI-based predictions of outcomes or AI-based recommendations for interventions, thus allowing the technology to claim a patient's decision-making power. For instance, let us say an AI system advises discontinuing life-sustaining treatment on a patient, when families or patients might just abandon the AE without really understanding what they are doing. It is only proper that this technology is controlled in a manner that respects patients' autonomy because there is a need to think through how such systems are made to be part of the decision-making process. Yet AI systems should be used to complement, not substitute, human judgement and patient input [50].

6.4 Decision-making and accountability

Making complex medical decisions at the end of life may be assisted by AI systems but the question of accountability follows in their wake. Who is responsible if the decision is wrong or if it is an incorrect prognosis or if a certain treatment is no longer required prematurely? Ultimately, medical decisions should be the responsibility of the ethically and legally responsible healthcare provider, acting in the best interest of his patient. But if an AI system suggests something that causes harm or makes a decision contrary to the wishes of the patient, it will be hard to know who is to blame. In addition, using AI in the care of the end of life increases the risk of algorithmic bias. If the AI system is trained on biased or non-representative data, it will provide either bad or biased recommendations. This could result in different communities receiving disproportionate care at the end of life and inequitable care which is disproportionately affecting certain demographic groups [51].

6.5 Human compassion vs. technological detachment

An additional ethical concern is that AI may take over where human compassion fails as regards care at the end of life. This is an intensely human thing to die, and friendly, compassionate, empathetic healthcare professionals are a critical part of helping relieve the pain of the patient and their families. But AI is, fundamentally, separated, and it does not have the emotional soup of human caregivers. Despite the ability of AI systems to simulate empathy through natural language processing or voice interactions, none of that is the same as having that human connection in a similar sensitive time [52]. It is a major ethical risk that we might get too dependent on technology to depersonalize the end-of-life experience. However, if AI is the primary means of handling end-of-life care, patients may feel alienated or de humanized if there is no human presence. Additionally, the use of AI could defeat the emotional support that family members and loved ones might feel, predisposing that the technology is taking over the responsibility of delivering care [53].

6.6 Equity and access

The integration of AI in end-of-life care alarms regarding equity and access to care. Like any technology, there is a chance that AI-powered solutions are only accessible to certain types of patients, that is, those in wealthier or more technologically advanced areas [54]. AI-based healthcare access may be lacking for marginalized or low-income communities, which adds to gaps in existing disparities in end-of-life care. To avert exacerbating social and healthcare inequalities, access to AI-driven end-of-life care solutions will remain a crucial step to be taken. Furthermore, the introduction of AI in the end of life in healthcare could redirect healthcare resources from humane solutions to technological solutions. In contexts where resources are already scarce, there is a tendency to favor technological solutions over human-centred care to the detriment of already marginalized populations [55].

7. Conclusion

Artificial Intelligence (AI) is undeniably transforming the landscape of modern medicine, including personalized medicine, genetic engineering, and end-of-life care. These advances hold the promise of improving patient outcomes, enhancing the efficiency of healthcare systems, and offering solutions to previously unsolvable challenges. However, while AI's potential is vast, its implementation also raises critical ethical, legal, and social questions that must be addressed carefully to ensure that its benefits are maximized while its risks are mitigated [56].

Today, in personalized medicine, the ability of AI to process vast amounts of data (including genetic info and epidemiological factors) has gained new capacity in precision healthcare. Glyceroneurometabolomics can predict how a patient is likely going to respond to a variety of treatments based on their genetically and molecularly unique profile, enabling personalized interventions with the highest efficacy and least adverse effects. In this context, the use of AI promises immense improvement in patient outcomes with complex or rare conditions where traditional "one size fits all" approaches often fall short [57]. Although personalization, like we know it now, can come with ethical concerns. But one big thing is genetic privacy protection. With such reliance on genetic data—and the accompanying risk of data breaches and misuse, including genetic discrimination by insurers or employers [7], the right rather crucial development is the establishment of a regulatory infrastructure that drives automation in genetic awareness. Additionally, while AI can infer how well treatments will work, algorithmic decision-making without adequate patient inputs or understanding could demote patient autonomy. Ultimately, AI-driven personalized treatments are further exasperating the potential for healthcare disparities; wealthier populations potentially benefit, while disadvantaged groups are at risk of falling behind [58].

Over the years, one of the most exciting uses of AI in modern science is that of genetic engineering, especially through tools such as CRISPR. Gene editing designs can be optimized by AI, predicted to have off-target effects, and analyzed against the massive genomic data needed for intervention. In theory, these technologies could eliminate inherited diseases, strengthen crop resilience and improve our human traits [59]. Despite the ethical importance of AI-driven genetic engineering, it still remains untested and contentious. Several ethical issues arise in what is known as germline editing: genetic modification in human embryos or reproduction cells, for example, to what degree should we interfere with human evolution? Nobody would want a genetically modified child programmed with certain desired traits; for instance, who would want a "designer baby", a child genetically modified for those "desirable" traits, at least it is the case that this creates further worries over inequality, consent, and the creation of a society prioritizing certain traits to the detriment of others [60]. In addition, there is the possibility of unintended, long-term consequences at the individual and human gene pool level. While better at genetic editing, AI also raises fresh fears of human capacity to control genetics and the risk of misuses like biohacking or engineering genetically altered organisms that in turn might have devastating ecological or societal harm [61].

There is plenty of promise in AI in end-of-life care. But AI systems are also being used to predict when patients will die, making it easier to plan effective palliative care. They can measure real-time health data, assist with symptom management such as pain and nausea, and offer clinicians tailored advice regarding care by decision-making. Early on, AI may also be used to provide emotional support, such as with virtual companions or robots, if human contact is not possible in such cases as joins of the healthcare system or pandemics (as in the case of COVID-19) [1]. However, all of these benefits raise significant ethical issues in regard to AI being used in end-of-life care. When automation of decision-making, particularly decision-making about life-sustaining treatments, fails to fully reflect patient or family wishes, the process undermines patient autonomy. Continuing with the above example, if an AI proposes withdrawing life support based on predictive analytics, the deeper ethical, and emotional factors in the decision-making process that humans' clinicians and family members bring to the decision are bypassed [62]. Additionally, reliance on AI for tasks that are so sensitive could counterproductively diminish the quality of compassionate care that is, after all, so often an important part of the end-of-life experience. It is important, therefore, to ensure that AI does not become a tool to replace, rather than a tool to support, human judgement in the dying process.

AI applications in medicine, notably in personalized medicine, genetic engineering, and end-of-life care, all demand robust ethical boarding for safeguarding patient rights. But it is also accountability, because AI systems are far from being infallible: they can make recommendations, but errors in decision-making have devastating results. What happens when AI systems get it wrong, making wrong predictions or recommendations? Who really is to blame for the mistakes: the AI tech developers, the clinician users of the tech or the patients who may not fully understand the tech? Decisions must be made with human responsibility at the centre, and there are clear guidelines needed. Another key point here on ethics is transparency. The decision-making of many AI algorithms follows "black boxes", the end users, such as the clinicians and patients, cannot easily understand the algorithms' inner workings. The absence of transparency can have an impact on the trust the communities have in these kinds of systems, in particular in high-stakes areas such as health care. If AI is going be used ethically, it needs to be both transparent and explainable for healthcare providers and patients to know how decisions are made and why specific recommendations are issued. If AI-driven healthcare solutions are to be an equitable system, this may be one of the most pressing ethical challenges. As the availability of these technologies grows within the health sphere, there is potential for the existing health inequalities to be compounded if they are only available to populations with the capacity to afford them (e.g., a high-income or high-wealth country) or as applied in the context of personalized medicine and genetic engineering. Closing the digital divide and ensuring that AI gains are achieved across all people, irrespective of their social and economic background, is important to enable these technologies to contribute to greater global health equity.

8. Final thoughts

As part of the AI Revolution happening right now, modern medicine is transforming today, including personalized treatments, genetic modifications and end-of-life care. Yet these technological advances need to be taken cautiously and with good judgment because they may infringe on the rights of the patient, their dependability and their "dignity". The goal is to use AI to increase healthcare outcomes while still embracing the core of the medical profession: it is deeply human. Finally, as we embrace AI in medicine, constant talk, regulation, and ethical standards need to be put in place to make sure that AI truly serves as a wonderful enabler in the healthcare field, that it makes healthcare this in a way that is equitable, kind and in sync with values of society.

Acknowledgements

The author acknowledges the usage of Google Gemini and Microsoft Copilot for language polishing of the manuscript.

Author details

Praveen Kumar Pradhan
GMCH, Sundargarh, Odisha, India

*Address all correspondence to: drpradhanpk@gmail.com

IntechOpen

References

[1] Iniesta I. Hippocratic Corpus. BMJ. 2011;**342**:d688. DOI: 10.1136/bmj.d688

[2] Jonsen AR. A Short History of Medical Ethics. USA: Oxford University Press; 2000

[3] Porter R. The Greatest Benefit to Mankind: A Medical History of Humanity from Antiquity to the Present. New York: HarperCollins; 1997

[4] Gillon R. Philosophical medical ethics. British Medical Journal (Clinical Research Edition). 1986;**292**(6519):111-113. DOI: 10.1136/bmj.292.6519.111

[5] Faden RR, Beauchamp TL. A history and theory of informed concsent. New York and Oxford: Oxford University Press; 1986

[6] Veatch RM. Disrupted Dialogue: Medical Ethics and the Collapse of Physician-Humanist Communication (1770-1980). New York and Oxford: Oxford University Press; 2005

[7] Pellegrino ED. Professionalism, profession, and the virtues of the good physician. Mount Sinai Journal of Medicine. 2006;**73**(3):377-384

[8] Mesko B. The role of artificial intelligence in precision medicine. Expert Review of Precision Medicine and Drug Development. 2021;**6**(1):5-8. DOI: 10.1080/23808993.2021.1885434

[9] Begoli E, Bhattacharya T, Kusnezov D. The need for uncertainty quantification in machine-assisted medical decision making. Nature Machine Intelligence. 2019;**1**(1):20-23. DOI: 10.1038/s42256-018-0004-1

[10] Rajkomar A, Dean J, Kohane I. Machine learning in medicine. The New England Journal of Medicine. 2019;**380**(14):1347-1358. DOI: 10.1056/NEJMra1814259

[11] Voigt P, Von Dem Bussche A. The EU General Data Protection Regulation (GDPR) [Internet]. Springer eBooks; 2017. DOI: 10.1007/978-3-319-57959-7

[12] Krittanawong C, Zhang H, Wang Z, Aydar M, Kitai T. Artificial intelligence in precision cardiovascular medicine. Journal of the American College of Cardiology. 2017;**69**(21):2657-2664. DOI: 10.1016/j.jacc.2017.03.571

[13] Wynants L, Van Calster B, Collins GS, Riley RD, Heinze G, Schuit E, et al. Prediction models for diagnosis and prognosis of COVID-19 infection: Systematic review and critical appraisal. BMJ. 2020;**369**:m1328. DOI: 10.1136/bmj.m1328

[14] Luxton DD. Recommendations for the ethical use and design of artificial intelligent care providers. Artificial Intelligence in Medicine. 2016;**62**:1-10. DOI: 10.1016/j.artmed.2014.12.004

[15] Ahmed Z, Mohamed K, Zeeshan S, Dong X. Artificial intelligence with multi-functional machine learning platform development for better healthcare and precision medicine. Database. 2020;**2020**:baaa010. DOI: 10.1093/database/baaa010

[16] Ahuja AS. The impact of artificial intelligence in medicine on the future role of the physician. PeerJ. 2019;**7**:e7702. DOI: 10.7717/peerj.7702

[17] Chen M, Decary M, Malczewska M. Ethical challenges of AI in personalized medicine: The case of AI-assisted cancer diagnostics. Frontiers in

Artificial Intelligence. 2021;**4**:563899. DOI: 10.3389/frai.2021.563899

[18] Li X, Dunn J, Salins D, Zhou G, Zhou W, Schüssler-Fiorenza Rose SM, et al. Digital health: Tracking physiomes and activity using wearable biosensors reveals useful health-related information. PLoS Biology. 2017;**15**(1):e2001402. DOI: 10.1371/journal.pbio.2001402

[19] Char DS, Shah NH, Magnus D. Implementing machine learning in health care—Addressing ethical challenges. New England Journal of Medicine. 2018;**378**(11):981-983. DOI: 10.1056/NEJMp1714229

[20] Binns S. Artificial intelligence and the ethics of gene editing. Bioethics. 2020;**34**(6):615-626. DOI: 10.1111/bioe.12822

[21] Cyranoski D. The ethics of editing the human genome. Nature. 2021;**590**(7846):324-328. DOI: 10.1038/d41586-020-00215-x

[22] Challen R et al. Artificial intelligence in health care: Anticipating challenges to ethics, governance, and regulation. Journal of Health Ethics. 2019;**14**(1):1-12. DOI: 10.1177/0020731420900186

[23] Kovacs G, Haeusermann R. CRISPR, ethics, and the future of genetic engineering. Genomics. 2020;**112**(3):345-355. DOI: 10.1016/j.ygeno.2020.03.007

[24] Lloyd H, Whitworth M. Ethical and social implications of artificial intelligence in personalized medicine. Ethics, Medicine and Public Health. 2020;**13**:99-105. DOI: 10.1016/j.jemep.2020.03.004

[25] Makino T et al. The role of artificial intelligence in genetic engineering and medicine: Opportunities and ethical concerns. Trends in Genetics.

2021;**37**(2):117-129. DOI: 10.1016/j.tig.2020.11.003

[26] Nuffield Council on Bioethics. Genome Editing: An Ethical Review. London: Nuffield Council on Bioethics; 2016

[27] Snyder M, Reddy S. AI and the ethics of personalized medicine: Towards a framework for responsibility. Artificial Intelligence in Medicine. 2021;**121**:103243. DOI: 10.1016/j.artmed.2021.103243

[28] Tellez D, Dillenburg H. Understanding bias in AI: Implications for the field of genetics. Journal of AI Research. 2020;**68**:125-142. DOI: 10.1613/jair.1.11893

[29] Wendler D, Rackoff J. Ethical challenges in AI-driven genetics: A global perspective. The Lancet. 2020;**395**(10231):937-939. DOI: 10.1016/S0140-6736(20)30256-1

[30] Doudna JA, Charpentier E. The new frontier of genome editing with CRISPR-Cas9. Science. 2014;**346**(6213):1258096. DOI: 10.1126/science.1258096

[31] Rasmussen LM, Friese MA. Ethical considerations in CRISPR-Cas9 gene editing and artificial intelligence in genetic medicine. Frontiers in Bioengineering and Biotechnology. 2020;**8**:422. DOI: 10.3389/fbioe.2020.00422

[32] London AJ. Artificial intelligence and black-box medical decisions: Accuracy versus explainability. Hastings Center Report. 2019;**49**(1):15-21. DOI: 10.1002/hast.973

[33] Challen R, Denny J, Pitt M, Gompels L, Edwards T, Tsaneva-Atanasova K. Artificial intelligence, bias and clinical safety. BMJ Quality &

Safety. 2019;**28**(3):231-237. DOI: 10.1136/bmjqs-2018-008370

[34] Topol EJ. High-performance medicine: The convergence of human and artificial intelligence. Nature Medicine. 2019;**25**(1):44-56. DOI: 10.1038/s41591-018-0300-7

[35] Obermeyer Z, Powers B, Vogeli C, Mullainathan S. Dissecting racial bias in an algorithm used to manage the health of populations. Science. 2019;**366**(6464):447-453. DOI: 10.1126/science.aax2342

[36] López D, Cheng R. Implications of Artificial Intelligence on Ethical Standards in Genetics and Biotechnology. New York: Genetic Engineering and Biotechnology News (GEN); 2019. Available from: https://www.genengnews.com/

[37] Glover J. Genetic engineering and the ethics of AI: A global challenge. Ethics and Technology. 2018;**16**(2):101-113. DOI: 10.1007/s10676-018-9472-0

[38] Turing AM. Computing machinery and intelligence. Mind. 1950;**59**(236):433-460. DOI: 10.1093/mind/LIX.236.433

[39] Price WN, Cohen IG. Privacy in the age of medical big data. Nature Medicine. 2019;**25**(1):37-43. DOI: 10.1038/s41591-018-0272-7

[40] Wicks P, Chiauzzi E. "Trust but verify" - five approaches to ensure safe medical AI. Journal of Medical Internet Research. 2015;**17**(5):e106. DOI: 10.2196/jmir.4352

[41] Mittelstadt BD, Allo P, Taddeo M, Wachter S, Floridi L. The ethics of algorithms: Mapping the debate. Big Data & Society. 2016;**3**(2):205395171667967. DOI: 10.1177/2053951716679673

[42] Leopold C, Chambers JD, Wagner AK. Access to AI-based personalized medicine: Ethical and equity considerations. The Lancet Digital Health. 2021;**3**(3):e142-e148. DOI: 10.1016/S2589-7500(20)30290-2

[43] Gómez E, Hall DM. Ethical issues in human germline editing and AI-assisted genomic technologies. Bioethics. 2021;**35**(3):239-246. DOI: 10.1111/bioe.12961

[44] Buchanan A, Brock DW. Bioethics and the regulation of genetic engineering: An ethical perspective on AI and human genetic engineering. Journal of Medical Ethics. 2021;**47**(4):252-259. DOI: 10.1136/medethics-2020-106424

[45] Nadimpalli M. Exploring AI's role in precision medicine: Gene editing and the future of healthcare. International Journal of Medical Informatics. 2020;**141**:104184. DOI: 10.1016/j.ijmedinf.2020.104184

[46] Dierckx M, Van den Noortgate W. The role of AI in end-of-life care: Ethical and practical challenges. Journal of Clinical Ethics. 2021;**32**(2):112-119

[47] He J, Wu Z. AI in healthcare: The ethical implications of using AI in end-of-life decision-making. Journal of Bioethical Inquiry. 2020;**17**(4):653-664. DOI: 10.1007/s11673-020-10055-1

[48] Shulman E, Cresswell K. Artificial intelligence and end-of-life care: The intersection of technology and human dignity. Ethics, Medicine, and Public Health. 2020;**14**:47-56. DOI: 10.1016/j.jemep.2020.04.005

[49] Sweeney M. The use of AI in palliative and end-of-life care: Challenges and ethical concerns. Journal of Palliative Medicine. 2019;**22**(9):1033-1039. DOI: 10.1089/jpm.2019.0266

[50] Wright AM, Miller MD. AI-assisted decision making in end-of-life care: Ethical and legal considerations. Journal of Medical Ethics. 2021;**47**(8):499-506. DOI: 10.1136/medethics-2020-106354

[51] Friedrich M, Theisen M. Artificial intelligence in end-of-life care: A systematic review of ethical issues. Palliative Medicine. 2021;**35**(6):943-949. DOI: 10.1177/02692163211000945

[52] Shulman L, Saldaña A. Exploring the role of artificial intelligence in end-of-life care: Implications for clinical practice and ethical responsibility. Journal of Palliative Care. 2020;**36**(4):283-290. DOI: 10.1177/0825859720940554

[53] Sutton J, Forlini C. AI and the ethics of predictive tools in end-of-life care. Journal of Clinical Ethics. 2020;**31**(3):345-354. DOI: 10.1080/13648470.2020.1751327

[54] Smith M, Clark R. Predictive analytics in end-of-life care: Opportunities and ethical challenges. Ethics, Medicine and Public Health. 2019;**9**:51-58. DOI: 10.1016/j.jemep.2019.01.005

[55] Gifford EM, Wu H. Humanizing end-of-life decisions: How artificial intelligence can enhance, not replace, compassionate care. Journal of Palliative Medicine. 2020;**23**(2):193-199. DOI: 10.1089/jpm.2019.0332

[56] Smith J. Artificial intelligence in medicine: Revolutionizing healthcare systems. Journal of Medical Innovation. 2023;**45**(2):67-80

[57] Johnson L, Lee M. AI and precision medicine: Personalized approaches to patient care. New Advances in Medical Technology. 2022;**31**(4):112-126

[58] Thompson B. Health disparities and the role of AI in personalized medicine. Journal of Health Equity. 2020;**22**(1):78-89

[59] Williams P, Zhang T. AI and genetic engineering: A new frontier in science. Molecular Biology Today. 2023;**28**(7):198-210

[60] Davis S. The ethics of germline editing: A case study on AI and CRISPR. Bioethics Quarterly. 2021;**35**(5):72-84

[61] Kaur R, Singh K. Risks of genetic modification: Ethical issues in AI-driven research. Biotechnology and Ethics. 2022;**17**(2):134-146

[62] Anderson N, Ramirez L. End-of-life decision-making: The impact of AI on human judgment. Journal of Ethical Medicine. 2023;**29**(4):77-91

www.ingramcontent.com/pod-product-compliance
Lightning Source LLC
Chambersburg PA
CBHW081336190326
41458CB00018B/6016